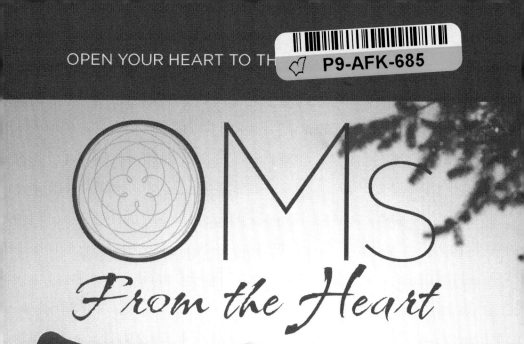

OMs
From the Heart

FLOWER OF LIFE
PRESS

Voices of Transformation

OMS FROM THE HEART: *Open Your Heart to the Power of Yoga*

Copyright © 2015 Dana Damara Evolution , www.DanaDamara.com

Published by Flower of Life Press, www.FloweroflifePress.com

Book Design by Jane Ashley
Cover Photo by Isabella Layon
Interior Photo and back cover photo by Eli Zaturanski Photography

Library of Congress Cataloging-in-Publication Data is available on file.

ISBN-13: 978-1523254606

Printed in the United States of America

Dedication

To my lovely daughters Isabella and Ava,

I am honored that you picked me to be your mother. I never imagined myself being a mother when I was younger. Instead I thought I would travel the world with one bag and witness its majestic views from behind a camera lens.

The story of us reminds me of the story of Ganesha—how when his parents, Parvati and Shiva ask their two children to go around the world as many times as they can, Ganesha simply spirals around the two of them, recognizing that they are his Universe and his world.

I feel that way about the two of you. The most majestic views have been watching you walk, listening to you sing, experiencing your drama, holding you tight. My most magical experiences are those I have had with you in simple, daily life. That's not to say I revolve my entire being around you. But it does mean that my heart is in consistent orbit with you and you are my Universe… always.

Thank you for your wisdom, intuition, dedication and unconditional love that you share with this world. Thank you for all the times you have been such amazing team players and shown up in such a mature way. Thank you for all the times you have come and cuddled with me in bed reminding me of your precious existence. Thank you for all the times you have called me out when I have fallen into patterns. Thank you for the times you have reminded me to ground in truth and integrity. And thank you for the times you have reminded me about the power of unconditional love.

The road hasn't been easy and I'm sure we will end up on many more windy, bumpy roads together. I know it hasn't been "perfect" when you compare our lives to others, but I can tell you this—it has been perfect. Perfectly imperfect.

There is one thing you can be sure of, my loves… I will always be here for you, no matter what. I will always tell you the truth, no matter what. And I will love you from the deepest recesses of my heart, even when it doesn't seem that way.

I believe that my most Divine calling in this life is to be your mother and I take my job seriously. One thing I ask from you: keep me laughing, dancing, and loving.

These Oms are for you.

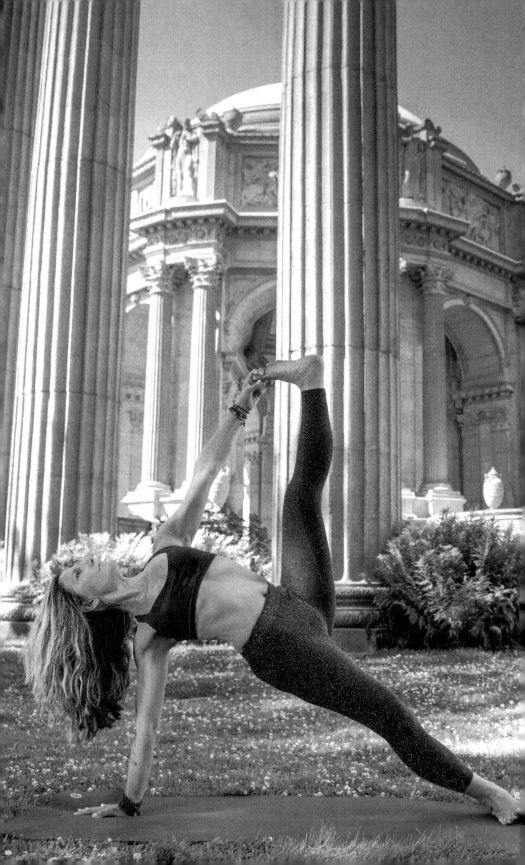

Contents

Acknowledgments

This book, *Oms from the Heart*, is a compilation of spiritual inquiries born from my dedication to connecting to the Divine. Once I began moving my body on my mat, my life came into focus. That is what birthed *Oms from the Mat*.

However, *Oms from the Heart* is different. Once I saw past the density of my being, witnessed my patterns, and peeled back a layer of stagnation, I remembered the light that lived within me and my heart began speaking in a big way. I was also receiving daily downloads of spiritual insight that propelled me into the most profound experience of growth in my life to date.

What I know to be true is this: beyond the stagnation there is deep unconditional love—always. Behind the patterns and projection there is acceptance and a remembrance that we are all truly One. And beneath the surface of the mind is an intuitive knowing and guidance.

All of this shows up through dreams, readings, teachings, and people. I want to thank a few of my most recent teachers for assisting in the creation of this book by just being in my life.

TJ—thank you for your amazing depth and connection to Source. And I must equally thank you for your perfectly imperfect human existence. For all the times you brought me to my knees in truth. Your questions rarely made me feel comfortable, but always offered such a potent message. Thank you for being my mirror of discontent, anger and fear of intimacy. And at the same time, thank you for being my mirror of unconditional love, deep passion, and connection to the Divine.

To my lovely teacher *Janet Stone*. You not only breathe love into all that you touch... you resonate truth and possess a Durga-like presence that has supported my dedication to this practice without you even knowing it. Your mothering is an example I follow in all of its exuberance, awe, and drama. Whenever I am at a crossroads, I ask, "What would Janet do?" Thank God you ask, "What would Beyonce do!" I am in good hands, my friend.

Thank you *Elayne Kalila Doughty*. Your presence has reminded me time and time again that this deep well of my being is infinite. That I am always supported and loved, and that there is always only one person in the room. You are the Gatekeeper of the Temple, and my life and expansion of my heart would not be the same without your grounding guidance and willingness to be transparent and vulnerable. You are such an important teacher in my life.

To my *mother* – for not always being there in a way I thought I wanted but always in a way that I needed. I see you—I *so* see you now. After surviving so many tumultuous times in my life recently, you have held such grace and presence, as any Goddess would. I love you so much.

And as one of my Beloved teachers says, "Make sure you're not giving too much power away and remember to acknowledge your role, too." So, I thank myself; for my own perseverance and commitment to truth, for continuing to open my heart when it was hurting, for standing in my stuff and loving it all. For walking a path I had talked about for years.

> *Guru Brahma, Guru Vishnu, Guru devo Maheshwara,*
> *Guru Sakshat, Param Brahma, Tasmai shri guravay namah*

> Our creation is that guru (*Brahma*—the force of creation); the duration of our lives is that guru (*Vishnu*—the force of preservation); our trials, tribulations, illnesses, calamities and the death of the body is that guru (*devo Maheshwara*—the force of destruction or transformation). There is a guru nearby (*Guru Sakshat*) and a guru that is beyond the beyond (*param Brahma*). I make my offering (*tasmai*) to the beautiful (*shri*) remover of my darkness, my ignorance; (*Guru*) it is to you I bow and lay down my life (*namah*).

With enormous amounts of gratitude I offer you *Oms from the Heart: Open Your Heart to the Power of Yoga*. Thank you for taking this journey with me.

Note from the Author

DANA DAMARA

In 2011 I made a hard right turn from comfortable life to the unknown. I left all my valuables and headed for the hills.

Literally.

It was several years after stepping on my yoga mat and consequently becoming awake to my life. I realized that my life was not the life I had envisioned and it was time for a re-birth. The hard work had been done, though—the Band-Aid had been ripped off and exposed all my wounds. I was ready for deep healing and it was time.

I packed it all up and left the Northwest for a new life in Northern California. *Oms from the Mat* reflects that journey and how I got there. It brought me through the fear, the guilt, the rage and the agony. The devotionals in *Oms from the Mat* were written from a place that would come into focus every time I stepped onto my mat, moved my body and cleared the stagnant energy of years past.

Oms from the Heart, however, is a bit different. It's written from the heart—truly. Yes, they are devotionals. They are written from the higher connection to Source I write about in *Oms from the Mat.*

After hitting the restart button on my life, I became more in tune with what was going on in my heart—what was evolving within my soul. My soul had been waiting so long to speak, and now that it had the chance, it wasn't wasting any time.

The devotionals in *Oms from the Heart* have a depth that is connected to the cosmos, to energy, and to the deep recesses of the heart. In the upheaval of my life, I found so many jewels—too many to count. One is my love for

Goddess energy and how potent it is. Another is my fascination with astrology and how it affects the body. Another is relationship and how deep our connections run if we are open to recognizing the Oneness in all things.

That is *Oms from the Heart*. The everyday reader will find resonance with the book on any given day, with any given Om. The yoga teacher can use the devotionals as a guideline or theme for classes.

Open the book, find the Om that speaks to you and "viola!" you have a theme for a class.

My hope is that anyone, yogi or otherwise, will pick this up and find something that resonates and speaks to their heart. Because the truth is, not everyone gets into the practice of yoga. It changed my life but it needn't be *your* catalyst. I ask you though, what IS your catalyst? What motivates you to observe and make a shift? And if not now, when?

My deep prayer for this book IS that it is used by yogis and yoga studios as a guide and in yoga teacher training programs, not only for theming classes but also to motivate other yogis to get out their pen and start writing.

My wish is that this book be a reminder for us all that we are more than we think we are.

We are always more.

8/23 the
Embody the
infinite presence
of magic within

Foreword

JANE ASHLEY, *Publisher*
December 2015

Meeting Dana Damara wasn't just a casual thing, though that was what I expected. I talk to people all day, and though I meet lots of cool and talented women, I didn't expect this call to inspire me the way it did. After we turned off Skype that afternoon, something was different—my energy was popping, and my imagination was flowing… I knew that I wanted to help this amazing woman spread her magic.

She sent me her first book, *Oms from the Mat*, and my publisher instinct was powerfully turned on! Wisdom and insight wrapped within wonderful writing—what gifts this little book held! I was excited to hear more, and Dana and I talked again…

Her journey since her book was published was full of the ups and downs that my tribe of conscious women have all experienced, and we talked about another book that went well beyond yoga, something that would speak to everyone.

Dana's work with women and girls has been transformative—powerful and full of her pure heart—a passion to serve, elevate, and create a safe space where truth is spoken and lives are transformed. The vision for her new book came together during that call, and the title we both loved adorns the cover of the book you are holding: *Oms from the Heart.*

Flower of Life Press is dedicated to bringing new and inspirational voices to the conversation, and I wanted to publish Dana's book for our list, and re-issue her first book at the same time.

What a fun ride we had! This woman is a powerhouse, make no mistake, and her goals are big. Books are but one facet of her essence—a way to express her truth and offer her deepest secrets to women of all ages.

Why do I find Dana Damara so inspiring?

It's very simple: She walks her talk. As a mom to two growing girls, she has a front-row seat, witnessing the challenges kids face in our discordant, totally wired world.

Not content with simply guiding her children, she created Girls Elevate™, a non-profit dedicated to building girls' self-esteem—creating connection between parent and daughter—and healing the planet through selfless service (SEVA) and community outreach.

With three teenage girls of my own, I witness the challenges girls face first-hand… and I honor Dana for stepping forward and leaning in, a leader unafraid to engage and show girls a different way to interface with this often confusing world.

As publisher, I am excited to be part of the movement Dana is building. As a woman dedicated to conscious conversation and the power of evolution, *Oms from the Heart* rocks my world!

Dana Damara is the real thing, a Priestess of the new paradigm, leading us all to the highest vibration, connecting Spirit and Soul within the hearts of women who desperately need to hear what she has to say.

Thank you for buying this book. Your life will change from reading it.

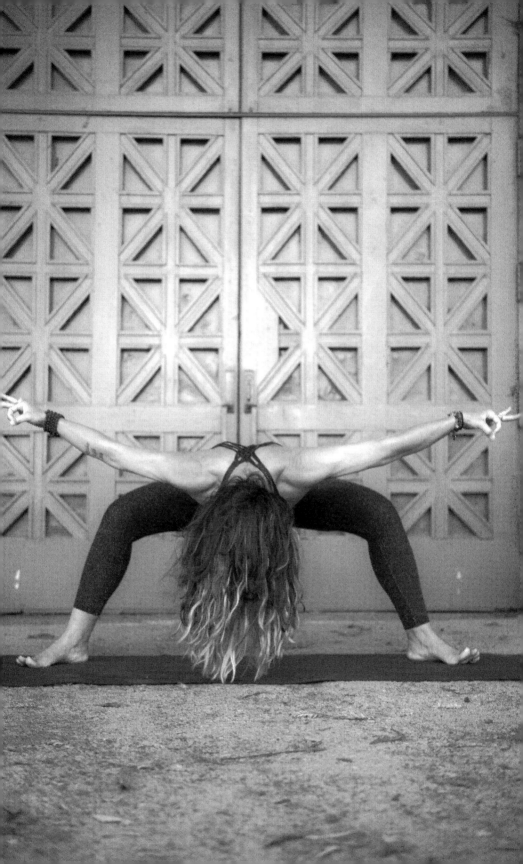

CHAPTER 1

On Grounding
Muladhara Chakra

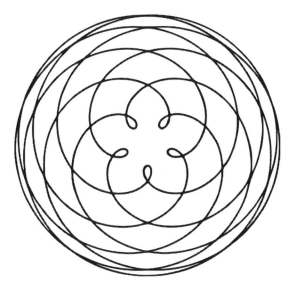

Alignment

The very first yoga class I ever attended was Iyengar based. This was some fifteen years ago, when I was totally into Tai Bo, Spin and Step Aerobics. Kind of an unusual transition, really. Truth be told, I hated it. I could hear the clock ticking, I did not sweat, and there was no music. It felt like such a waste of time to me. It took me a good month to go back. Honestly, it was like pulling teeth, but something kept me going back once a week.

It was the alignment... the alignment kept me safe in all the other things I was doing with my body. My risk of injury decreased because I really started focusing in on what my body was actually doing and where my limitations were. I started looking at my body as a skeleton and inherently knew when it was in alignment and when it was not.

This is where the yoga begins, with the body. Our humanity gazes at our physical presence first because that is how we relate in the world. Iyengar put it this way:

> *"We begin the involution with what is most tangible, our physical body, and the yogasana practice helps us to understand and learn how to play this magnificent instrument that each of us has been given."*

This is truth... so we start there. He has also mentioned that many people come to yoga because of dis-ease in the body. They are hurting and in pain and do not know why. He says,

> *"Health begins with firmness in the body, deepens to emotional stability, then leads to intellectual clarity, wisdom and finally the unveiling of the soul." And, "A yogi never forgets that health must begin with the body. Your body is the child of the soul."*

This man was a sage living among us, and when I read his book *Light on Life*, my life changed. My perspective changed; my world shifted.

With regard to pain, he also said,

"It is not the yoga that causes the pain, the pain is already there. It is hidden. We just live with it or have learned not to be aware of it. It is as if the body is in a coma. When you begin yoga, the unrecognized pain comes to the surface."

I overflow with gratitude for this man's gift of wisdom, practicality and grace. Because of his teaching, I am able to share with my students a powerful flow that will keep them safe and in alignment with their bodies. They experience the breath so their mind can be clear. And they can begin witnessing themselves from a place of compassionate observation.

But more than that... if we can remember this: *Our body is a reflection of our mind and our soul. The intention of yoga is to get the body, mind and soul all in alignment so we can live our deepest truth. The word* yoga *means "to yoke" or to "unite" so how could it be any other way?*

Iyengar, I bow to you, as do many others. Your legacy of love and light will live on forever. I am grateful for your teaching as it carries us all through life with a beacon of connection, strength and depth.

Infinite rounds of *Om*...

Commitment

I wrote about this in my book *Oms from the Mat,* and when I re-read it this past week, it made even more sense to me.

I said something like, "If commitment is such a strong word, I wonder why we sometimes use it so loosely." And then I went on to say, "Even if you have to just pick one thing... pick it and be committed to it! No matter what it is... a yoga class, a person, your word, just do it!"

Since moving to California in November 2012, nothing has rang more true to me in my life. Nothing.

Amidst the most AMAZING opportunities of this big move... (and I mean it... magic occurs every single day), I have also experienced mass confusion, dead-ends, fearful situations, lonely times and deep pain.

Betcha didn't know that did you? Well, it's true.

What I have found through all of this is that I have one strong commitment that has kept me going. There have been times when I have wanted to give up, run back to Portland and cuddle next to a fire with a friend... claiming "safe."

That would be easy to do any day of the week, given that I have amazing friends in the Northwest. But I haven't. I've been committed and dedicated to my practice. And I'm not talking about my practice on the mat. I'm not talking about my sequencing or playlists, although they do play an important role.

And oddly, I'm not talking about the commitment I made to my two amazing daughters either. No, that's not the commitment I am talking about. I am talking about the commitment I made to myself to live my truth. Because I know as well as you do that truth=freedom=love.

When we make a commitment to ourselves, we may THINK it's about: making money for our family, showing up our best for our students, helping the planet, serving our employer... but it's not any of that. It's about YOU.

The evolution of YOU and how YOU grow and elevate your spiritual being.

It's super easy to give up just before that breakthrough. You know what I am talking about, right? It's that last straw, that final argument, the repeating dead-end. It's that moment when you scream and say, "That's it! I give! That's it! I'm done!"

Have you ever done that? My suggestion to you from personal experience, having said those words in my life more than I care to admit, is to instead... breathe and keep going. You are almost there.

Now I'm not saying keep on taking what isn't working. What I am saying is *notice*. Observe what is happening in as many exchanges as possible.

When you feel that recurring uncomfortable knot in your stomach, or tightness in your throat, breathe. Maybe you just feel "off." Use the element of the heart and breathe into the belly. Root into your feet and feel it all... if only for five breaths. Then ask, what can you do differently in this situation, instead of walking away? What can you commit to right now that will keep you on the path of self-evolution?

Is it patience? Compassion? Trust? Love? Self-love? Knowing what it is that YOU, your soul, is working on to grow is key here. Once you get that, oh my, you will see so many circumstances coming up for you that will assist in your dedication and commitment to moving past it. It might feel like you are getting a bit bombarded to be honest, but you will be okay... once you know it's all there to help you.

We all have recurring issues or stories. Before you keep telling the same story over and over again, keep quiet and observe. Commit to rolling through it differently... it's showing up for a reason. You called it in... mmmm hmmm.

Courage Creates

Whew... *courage*, what a word. I was told by one of my amazing teachers once that the word *courage* actually radiates the highest vibration when it comes to connecting with the Divine. That blew me away. One of the most powerful virtues, she said. Because it creates. It creates the next thing based on your decision to make a decision that best suits your development. If you are present, that is.

It doesn't mean you will make the "right" decision... it just means you will make one based on your heart perhaps and not the inner workings of your mind.

I believe courage happens in every moment. It happens when you leap forward into something that is unfamiliar. It happens when you relax in the familiar. It happens when you speak your mind and when you listen. It happens when you move forward and when you let go. It happens when you stand strong and when you open up to vulnerability.

Courage happens every moment of every day. Are you present to how courageous you are?

I was home with my oldest daughter this week so I had a lot of time to think. I couldn't focus on creating a whole lot while she had a fever so high that it made my skin crawl. So I had a ton of time to think about courage.

And of course I was offered a multitude of opportunities to stand in courage. To be honest, the thoughts started out as a pity party. "Oh my God, it takes courage to be a mom!" You know, pretending that you're not scared when you really are. "Keeping it all together" when really you are scared shitless... literally. Then it went to, "I'm falling into fear here, I have to call in for backup," meaning I called upon my lovely women friends who have the power to heal. And my other women friends who could help me out a bit.

Reaching out takes courage, you know.

The moment I reached out, I remembered that it takes courage to be a parent, not just a mom. And then immediately, almost before that thought ended, I remembered that it takes courage just to love. To love.

Courage to love.

What a concept. Yes... that is the courage of all courage.

To love what?

Another person. To trust them with your heart.

Your child. They will leave you, you know. They will go off and do their thing. Despite your dreams for them, they will do their own thing.

Yourself. Yes, it takes a huge amount of courage to stand in the mirror and love what you see. All of it, not just the good parts.

Your ex-partner (or someone else who may trigger you). Gotta love them too. They taught you something AND you loved them... a lot at one point.

Courage to love... to love it all and move with a grace and ease that is palpable. To step out on a limb without knowing what is going to happen. To put your heart out there not knowing how or if it will be received.

Courage to be present...

Yes... to be present to it all. To SEE it all from the view of your heart. To WITNESS it all with breath and a knowledge that nothing is yours except your heart and your reaction to life and love.

Now, got get 'em!

Courageous Soul

The theme courage came flying to me the moment I heard that the New Moon was in Aries and that Pluto had gone into retrograde.

Let me put it to you simply: opposing energies, both working in our benefit, both taking courage to harness.

Meaning, it takes courage to leap forward in life, like the fiery energy of Aries. And it takes courage to sit still and examine our stuff that has been shoved into the back corner of our closets (or under the rug), before leaping forward.

It takes courage to do it all.

I started contemplating it, and I think we display courage in every waking moment. I mean, we're courageous when we speak, we're courageous when we're silent. We are courageous when we try something new, and we're just as courageous when we sit and wait our turn.

I used to think that courage came from our will, our drive to move forward and follow our passions and... impulses. I used to think that it took courage to leap without thinking. And I used to think it took courage to stand for what you believe in and speak your mind.

I still believe that.

And I think it takes courage to sit and see what happens for a moment. And I think it takes a hell of a lot of courage to listen... especially when you may not like what you hear. It takes courage to expose your heart and be seen for who you truly are. And it takes courage to accept and unconditionally love those around you.

I used to think it took courage to live and stand in your power. Now I think it takes courage to live from your heart, to expose the truth of how you feel without expectation or attachment. To love without knowing how the other person feels. To let go not knowing what is next.

I came home from work tonight to some, you know, pre-teen drama. And I witnessed my daughter courageously admitting that she was wrong, saying how she felt and then taking responsibility for her actions from her heart on her SLEEVE!

The world NEEDS courageous hearts, those souls willing to SPILL IT, fall on their face, get back up and do it again. The world NEEDS more people willing to LOVE ALL OUT and go ALL IN, diving deep and coming back to the top refreshed and in reverence for it all, every, last bit.

Repeat after me... I am a courageous soul, I am a courageous soul, I am a courageous soul. Now go be that.

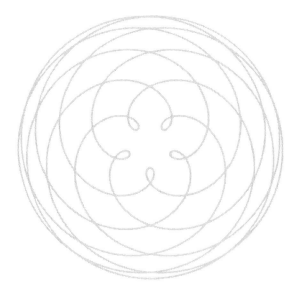

Epic Transition

On Friday, March 20, 2015, as the sun emerged from its deep sleep and moved into the Spring Equinox, it was obscured by a Solar Eclipse, creating opposing energies of forward motion and a sitting back and waiting. This isn't anything new, you know, movement forward, movement backward. This is what happens in transition. Even though an astrological event like this in the cosmos rarely happens, transitions certainly have their hiccups.

And when the stars align like this—New Moon, New Season, New Astrological calendar and a Solar Eclipse—I have to say that EPIC TRANSITION is the only theme that comes to mind.

This is indicative of transition, though, if you think about it. A little forward motion, a little reverb back to the old. It's called the human experience.

This was what I wrote: *The Spring Equinox happens around 3:45pm PST and it's coupled with an end of the astrological calendar, meaning we end at zero degrees Pisces and transition into Aries right around that same time, if I'm reading all of this correctly.*

Not only that, but we are coming off of a Pluto/Uranus, square meaning more transition and potentially a shift in energy that we've been sitting with since around October 2012. The Pisces New Moon/Solar Eclipse occurs at 2:36am PST on that same day, creating what I liken to a portal... a portal that you get to choose how you approach.

This is all about transitions, big ones at that. And I mean it. I do believe, though, that you can shift 2 degrees or 180 degrees; that you can create effort or ease; that you can struggle or flow. I believe that everything is a choice. However, we do not have the option to change or not; change is inevitable especially in times like this astrologically.

I believe that we are always transitioning—always evolving, always growing **and** we get to choose how that looks. With all of this epic movement happening out there, do you really think that YOU are exempt from that energy? Do you REALLY?

Newsflash: You're not.

So I've been asking myself, how do I want to enter into this new paradigm? Because that's what it is, you know. A completely new reality. And when we enter into transitions like this, it's not like we just sit down and intend our life. No, we have to really look at the whole ball of wax and ask ourselves what works and what doesn't. We must be willing to release the intense grip we have on the old so the new can come in. And, I believe that if we don't release it, the Universe is so powerful it's going to do it for us.

So, we have a choice as always. *Let go or be dragged. Up-level or stagnation.*

How will you embody these transitions? In your relationships? Your career? Your environment? Your finances?

If you can remember that everything happens in response to your perception and in favor of your evolution, transition cannot be anything but epic. So why fight it?

Fear, worry, doubt—all nonsense. Listen, if you're reading this and you think you have control of anything, take a look up at the sky. Figure out how the Moon makes waves. Tell me how Mars and Venus align and how all this epic shit happens on one day.

Tell me how all that alignment happens while you sleep!

Then settle into what is, buckle up, smile that smirky smile, and be present for the ride. Make it epic... because it always is!

Foundation

The other day, I'm in the car with my youngest daughter and she asks me, "Mom, is there an end to the sky?" And I said... "Um no honey. It's infinite." And she says... "Infinite... like energy?" And I say, "Yup, just like that." And she sat there for quite awhile looking up and out of the sunroof. As if she was trying to figure it all out.

We didn't talk that much after that but I could tell the wheels were turning.

It got me thinking about the word *foundation* and how daunting it can be. I mean, if the Earth is spinning and the sky is infinite, are we really standing on any type of foundation?

Yes, most certainly we are. Ourselves.

I contemplated foundation for a while before I wrote this. And I remembered a few times in my life when I had no physical foundation. Once when I was twenty-six and traveled to the South Pacific for an entire year—with one bag, no cell phone, no Internet. Once when I was working on yachts when I was about thirty-something. Every day was an adventure—waking up in a different port, different time zone and, sometimes, a different country. And then this last time, when I moved to California with no foundation except a job that paid pennies when I first started.

Foundation... security... stability—it is all an illusion if you look outside yourself for it. Foundation is an inside job and it is found only when you feel into the power that lives within you. It's found when you tap into your intuition and make decisions from there. It is recognized in tight situations, when the going gets rough. It is exemplified when you remember your foundation is your connection to Source, to God, to your internal compass.

And sometimes, that's all you have. But that's all you need. Ever.

From an outside, human perspective, it's easy to see how we can get swayed by things, or people, or jobs, or even homes to determine our foundation. But, I'm telling you... the only foundation you ever need is the one you have with yourself and with God, however you define God. To be quite honest, God has been defined many different ways throughout my life.

My foundation had been ripped out from underneath me several times in this life, and I believe it was an initiation to up-level my connection to Spirit and to my own intuitive knowing. We must be reminded in this life that we need nothing but ourselves... nothing but our truth... nothing but our heart.

I get it, it's challenging. I have two kids and I try to "create a foundation for them to feel safe and comfortable in." And, yes, I use those exact words. At the same time, they know it could change in a moment's notice and not to get too attached. Perceived foundation is a dangerous game. I'd rather connect deep into my physical body, my boundless heart, and my God-guided intuition. Those will never go away.

Grounded

Stability. What does it mean to you?

We are an interesting breed, we humans. Often we surround ourselves with things that make us feel secure in this ever-shifting world.

And we all do it. No one is exempt. We find a community to contribute to and lean on, a job to receive financial energy from, a home to root into and spread out our stuff in, a partner to "complete" us, and material items to call our own.

The funny thing is, when anything in that "stable environment" goes away, starts to crumble or falls apart, we turn to something to replace it with. Another community, another job, another home, another partner and more material items. We may even look to various healing modalities to get to the root of our issues.

While some of this can be temporarily helpful, the truth is we are multi-dimensional beings and we must search deeper for the answers we seek. But when change comes our way, we tend to go down the same path because we forget that we are spiritual beings living a human experience and, quite frankly, it's just easier to do the same thing over and over again.

No one is exempt... not even the most "enlightened" yogi. A few things I want to share with you as you embark on any transformative journey: (because you will if you haven't already... it's inevitable):

- You really DO create what you want. It's ALL about your perception of reality. So ask yourself... what DO you want?

You do get to pick. If you sit long enough, visualize clearly enough, write down your desires and then take those thoughts out into the world, it WILL come to you. And it will come to you swiftly. As swiftly as you allow it to, that is. AND depending upon how many times you block it with your past thoughts, behaviors and patterns. Maybe it's time to try something new.

- Before you step forward... look behind you.

Your past is important. Spend just enough time there to UNDERSTAND, or at the very least RECOGNIZE, your patterns of behavior. You can only manifest what you desire after you look at your patterns and realize that YOU are what is holding you back. No outside circumstance or person holds you back... it's all you. Trust me on this one. Same behavior equals same results.

- Understand that all these "things" that you surround yourself with do NOT hold the answers. The answers come in stillness. Period.

Just know that nothing, not one single material item, person, or perceived stable solution will move you forward. The ONLY way for forward motion to happen... forward motion into expansiveness, that is... is if you realize your strength is within. It's who you are. It's how you stand and how you breathe. It's how rooted you are, no matter what shows up for you on any given day, in any given moment.

So ask yourself... who are you? What do you stand for? Can you feel that internal strength and connection with all that IS root you into the Earth?

Here's how we play with this in yoga.

Bandhas... breath... internal gaze.

Allow your roots to dig deep beneath your feet. Notice that YOU root deep, all on your own. Feel your breath circulate through your body within that stable base and understand that that is the catalyst of forward motion... with a firm foundation. And then most of all... exercise that internal gaze.

Do not be fooled by external influences, thinking they will move you forward or keep you rooted. I can tell you, from experience... the BEST way to find your footing on this planet and your place in this world, is to strip it all away. Be with nothing... I mean it... nothing. Be with you and you alone. No community, no home, no job, no partner, no material items. Just you. If only in your mind... if only for a moment.

What will you find?

Once you get past the fear of being alone, not being accepted, hurt, or judged, and once you get past all those old voices telling you all those statements that mean nothing to you, you will find You. This amazing, strong, bright light that isn't clouded with fear, judgment, material items and old ideas. It's you... poised, ready and full of purpose, power and passion.

Manifest

I've done a lot of work and training around this word *manifest*. It continues to intrigue me and excite me, for sure. I mean it's such a simple word, right?

Manifest: *To make clear or evident to the eye or understanding. To create. To bring forth.*

But manifesting can be so challenging, can't it? You want to know why it's so challenging? Because we try too hard. We don't allow for the seed to take root and then show up at its own pace. We hurry it along and wait impatiently sometimes for "it" to show up when we feel it is time.

You see, most often when we "want" to manifest something, we say things like, "I want this" or "I want that." But what happens when we use the words *I want* or *I need*... It just creates more lack.

You see, the Universe likes to mirror itself. It can't wait to deliver to you what you desire. But you have to use the proper language. You must state it as if it is already present. You must feel it as if it is already yours. And then it will show up when it is time... and not a moment before.

It's planting a seed within us. The idea comes from the soul and it must be planted and then tended to. But with just the right amount of love, attention, intention and ambition... and not an ounce more. Because the other part to manifesting is allowing. Allowing the seed to sprout when it wants, and to grow at its own pace.

So we sit back and allow... and we trust... and we do our thing while manifestation happens behind the scenes.

You see, here's the deal... we are creating in every moment. Every thought we have starts the manifestation process. If that thought makes it out of your mouth and is verbalized, it's even more potent. And Goddess look out if you write it down... it's here. In some dimension, it's here. You just have to believe that and wait for it to show up.

And from what I have experienced... when we truly let go, when we completely allow, we are gifted with a miracle. One that our little brains could have never imagined. Not in a million years. So what do we do, then, to manifest?

State it... believe it... feel it and then allow it. Easy. You got this.

Manifestation

Sometimes I sit back and look at my life and I think, *Wow, I created this.* This is a far cry from where I used to be which was, *How did I get here?* The difference between the two thoughts is simple. One comes from a highly awakened state, and the other is from a very deep sleep.

The power of the mind is intriguing. I mean, to take on the responsibility of your life is slightly daunting, right? It is much easier to blame people, circumstance, environment and your ancestors for what shows up in your life, isn't it?

Let me ask you this: Do you believe that our life is predestined or do you think we have a hand in what transpires? What a thoughtful question to ask yourself at this time on the planet.

Personally, I believe we all show up with karma—an agenda if you will, that on a soul level, we want to clear. And this karma shows up throughout our lifetime (okay, lifetimes!). It presents itself as challenging situations, *risk-taking* opportunities, day-to-day activities, and conditions that blow our hearts wide open... pushing us to the depths of our being.

Now, we have a choice: We can let these situations blow by, chalking them up to coincidence, or we can breathe into them and witness the magic. We can point our finger outward or we can look inward and ask how we contributed to what is showing up and, even deeper, why we created it.

And you know, one way isn't right and one isn't wrong; it's just a matter of how deep you really want to go with all of this.

Ask yourself this question: "If I could be, do or contribute anything in this lifetime, without limits, what would it be?" First, notice how quickly the mind comes in with its limits and restrictions, listing the reasons why you can't be all that! It happens that fast... because, mostly, those limiting beliefs are unconscious and they race through your mind like wildfire.

Then ask yourself, "Is this idea or vision anywhere present in my life and, if it's not, why isn't it?" This usually sets off what I like to call the "snow-globe effect," where things start to be shaken up a bit. Nothing makes sense. However, underneath it all, it ALL makes sense; you are just waiting for everything to settle.

Because the truth is, we CAN create our lives. We DO create our lives. We ARE creating our lives. We are manifesting in every single moment of every single day. Our thoughts truly do create our reality. And what's funny is manifestation can happen in an instant or it can take some time. It's really dependent upon how much we feel into that thought; how much we believe that thought; and how much we are willing to clear from our life in order to allow that thought to manifest.

What happens when we look at our lives and ask, "How did I get here?" An avalanche of unconscious belief comes crashing down on us and is lying in a pile of rubble at our feet. What is underneath is who we have been all along, but it's seemingly new so it feels uncomfortable. It has been safe and comfortable, living underneath that pile of rubble. Because you didn't have be vulnerable, you didn't have to take responsibility, you didn't have to show your Self.

What I have found, over the past few years, though, is that once that initial avalanche falls, you feel... exposed. Life all of a sudden looks different. And, honestly, you never really go back to "how did I get here." You really don't.

You fall into the breath, slow-mo your life and feel it all. And in those moments, it is as if your life is flying across the ticker tape of your mind and you see all the choices you made that got you to that moment.

You realize that you did create the situation you are in. You understand the power of your mind and your heart harmonizing in creation. And you feel pure reverence. It's like time stands still and you witness that space... you SEE what choices you made, what thoughts you thought, what words you said and what you wrote in the privacy of your own journal that brought you right there... in that moment.

And this is all REGARDLESS of what the moment is. Because you can't attach to the moment. Not even for a second.

That is what usually throws people off... labeling the moment. Because if the ego comes in and labels the moment as good or bad, right or wrong, then the mind starts playing games... usually the blame game, which never ends on an enlightened note.

You've got to stay with the breath, that's the only way... and in the heart, which is where the breath lives anyway.

It never ceases to amaze me, blow my mind, or take my breath away— that acceptance of the power we possess. In an instant of being, when I am offered that space to notice, I am in full reverence for the pure magic of creation. In that long deep breath of awareness, I notice my words, my meditations and my vision boards. I see my circle of influence, my prayer, my heart, and I realize I am in union with God, creating my life.

You are an amazing manifester. What do you want to create?

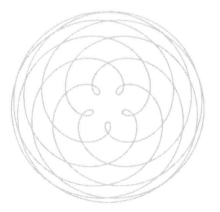

No More Coddling

When I first started teaching yoga, I remember wanting to be sure that EVERYONE could do the pose I was instructing. I learned to teach from a place that was inclusive to all. I love that about my very first teacher training. It taught me to go slow, to connect and to find empathy. It taught me to look at bodies from a new perspective every time I walked into the room.

That was several years ago, and I still teach like that. I think it serves the greater population not calling a class "Level 1" or "Level 2" but instead calling it something fun like Bohemian Flow, just to pique interest. Because, really, who the hell knows what level they are when it comes to yoga? I mean it. Unless you try, you will never know how far your body can go.

I think instead we keep it vague but genuine, and instruct class from a place that is grounded in deep foundation and complete attention to detail. Instead of getting hung up on the name of the class, we cultivate an awareness of our students' bodies and what is going on for them in these postures. This takes continued education, unwavering awareness, and a willingness to listen.

Now, having said that, I have something to add as far as teaching, sharing and leading a class, and this is important.

> *Yoga instructors: We must stop coddling our students if we want them to grow.* I mean, safety is important of course. But yoga is kinda like raising children... they have to fall if they are going to learn anything at all. They may hurt themselves on this journey, but it's not all your responsibility... they have to take some of it on as well.

Here are a few tips to keep it real along this practice of teacher-student and back again:

- Watch their bodies and teach them to listen to their own.

- Know stress is okay; it actually pushes one past a point of comfortable complacency.

- Start at the beginning, encourage private sessions or a Yoga 101 if necessary.

- Keep learning and sharing; they are hungry for expansion, whether they admit it or not.

Patience

A lot has been happening on this side of the screen, and honestly, I've had to have a lot of patience with myself while I traverse, once again, into some new skin.

Patience with my kids...

Patience with my "wusband"...

Patience with myself...

Patience with the process...

Patience while I listen intently to the Universe and its plans for me. To be quite honest, I've been sitting in the lap of abundance. But what I've found is that just because you're experiencing abundance does not mean that it's all right for you in this moment.

All my life I've wanted to know what's next. I've wanted to hurry to the next thing. And when an opportunity presented itself, I would think, "I better jump on this opportunity because, well, it's here for me to take it, right?"

No, not so much. Opportunities are not here for us to take. They are here for us to observe. To recognize their alignment with who we are in THIS moment. To sit with and feel into. To resonate or release.

What I've learned is that patience, when we really breathe into it, reveals the truth. I've also learned that sometimes, when an opportunity comes up, it's only there to show you an example of what's coming. And if you wait just a hot little minute, what's coming when you release that opportunity is much more magnificent than what you could have dreamed up.

You feel me on this one?

I remember, when I was younger, saying out loud, "I wish I could wiggle my nose and get to where I am supposed to be next." When I got older and I was going through a tough time, instead of dropping into the struggle, I would run away and move onto something else. So instead of having patience with the process and learning from the journey, I just wanted the destination or the end result.

What did that do? Re-create lesson after lesson after lesson until I finally woke up and recognized the pattern.

The pattern of thinking I knew it all.

The pattern of not-enoughness... I better grab THIS opportunity; another one might not come along.

The pattern of skimming the surface of my life for an illusion of perfection.

None of that works.

We don't know it all.

There are infinite opportunities and an abundance of resources.

The depth of our journey reveals our connection to the Divine.

Patience is not just a virtue. It is a pathway to the Divine.

It is the key to soulful living.

Patience is the recipe for truth, freedom and love.

We sit and we wait; we wait for the breath of the Divine to guide us into our truth and our purpose. We have patience as we observe our life and all the amazingness that happens as we move through each connection, each struggle, each embrace and each disappointment. We have patience, and when it's right and it's time... we know. That's all. We just know.

Resiliency

Resilience is a powerful tool in anything you are undertaking in your life. As always, I MUST bring these practices off the mat!

Resilience is defined as the ability to return to our original form after resistance. I would like to elaborate on that a bit and propose that resilience is *the potential to flow through resistance, witnessing instead a NEW version of a posture, a thought, a relationship. One that is stronger, full of more grace and wisdom.*

We all meet resistance, right? To be perfectly honest, we create the resistance on a subconscious level to become stronger. Sounds funny, but it's truth... believe me.

Our soul really wants us to evolve, and it keeps giving us situations that offer us the opportunity to move past the resistance WE created! Our mind is what gets in the way; our stories get in the way; our beliefs get in the way. I mean, it's safer to stay in the same habitual patterns of thought, words, and actions than it is to risk looking like a fool, right?

No one wants to fall on their face in *Vasisthasana*, especially next to the sexy girl (or guy) in class. No one wants to admit they don't know something. No one wants to put their heart out there, not knowing if the love will be returned.

But what if, just what if, we could move past that resistance, or that fear of falling, or of being ignorant, or that fear of loving, just to love without conditions or expectation? What would that build in us?

Oh, a power of self-love, authenticity, connection and inner strength that would speak volumes in this messy world. It would build us up, from the INSIDE OUT, offering us a chance to build endurance, balance and strength to move us further and expand us by opening our hearts.

On a global level, it would heal this world. It would bind us to our truth, our purpose. It would set us on a trajectory of KNOWING ourselves so well that everything that vibrated to us was ONLY there to serve us in our power to heal and elevate the planet. The Universe would respond in such a powerful way, all you would have to do is sit back and say, "Of course. I'm ready. May I have another please?"

All because you were willing to fall. You were willing to put yourself out there on a limb, without any attachment.

When we build that inner strength BASED ON our willingness to not know, to fall, and to love fully... we become so resilient that nothing, nothing knocks us down. And when we do get knocked down, we don't care! We just get up, dust off, smile and move forward. We become so focused on our inner eminence of Divine love, strength and connection that we can't help but continue in the flow of moving forward.

Resiliency is the power to return back to your original form after resistance. Side plank offers us the chance to build endurance, balance, and strength and then the chance to go farther by opening our hearts. When we meet our challenge, we then return back to our original form, finding ourselves more resilient than ever.

Start small... offer yourself up to falling in love. Admit you don't know something. Fall on your face... literally. You will then be liberated to show up authentic, ready to share your gifts, and THAT is what this world needs.

Sturdy and Steadfast

I've been watching this full moon and, to tell you the truth, I am so excited to work in this energy—grounding in and getting rooted! After all the upheaval, the transformation, the undeniable realigning... it's time to grow some roots and be devoted to my path.

These two words came so clearly to me and I wasn't even sure why until I looked them up. It's been a doozy, this energy that started all the way back in July 2015. Whether or not you get what I'm talking about is really just a matter of how much you've been paying attention. Or, more honestly, how much you've been willing to look at, shift, release, and accept this journey you call your life.

All I can really say about sturdy and steadfast is this: *We have been given quite a show, an amazing opportunity, if you will, to realign and redesign our lives. To live in our own vortex of truth, freedom and love. And to be free from the things that hold us back.*

We've been asked to live our dharma and burn through as much karma as we are willing to churn for the sake of liberation. And we've been asked to do this with a grace that is palpable, a heart that is open and a stance that is sturdy and righteous.

We've been asked to look at our life with a new lens that radiates from the soul instead of reflecting the past or someone else's vision and dreams. It's almost as if the Universe has come in and said, "Enough living in someone else's shadow. Enough playing small. And enough blaming everyone else around you. It is time to live in truth and stay there." As if our path has been carved out with clarity and direction and oh, by the way, all the resources you will need are here, on this path... you just need to trust and move toward it with sturdiness and devotion.

It's happening, and this full moon in Taurus is doing all sorts of collaborating with the Universe to make sure you stay the course.

My question is, *Where are you a bit wobbly? Where do you feel less than supported? Why? And if you are a bit wobbly but see the path clearly, why are you hesitating? What holds you back from following that course? What is distracting you? And how have you let this distraction come in again?* Because it's not the first time it has happened.

Now is the time to do something different. To stand grounded and sturdy. To move with a laser sharp intensity that is devoted to your truth, your freedom and your love. To stay off everyone else's path and follow your own.

Yes, your own.

It's time and I'm wondering—or hoping, rather—that you are ready.

Tribe

I've been thinking a lot about the word *tribe* over the past week. I just got back from my annual trip to Wanderlust in Squaw Valley, and that word simply encompasses how I feel the minute I step foot into that festival.

Tribe: *"Any aggregate of people united by ties of descent from a common ancestor, community of customs and traditions."*

My blood family raised me, and for that, I am beyond grateful. My yoga tribe, on the other hand, remembers me. The knowing of tribe members is unexplainable and may show up as synchronicities or mystical encounters. While I agree that some of us may feel that with our blood family, others do not. When I arrive at Wanderlust every year, I can't help but feel like I'm with my family.

We travel to each other and gather with a common interest and passion of making sustainable change with our various forms of art, music, dance and yoga. We know that when we come together, the energy creates a vortex that is mystical and magical. We know that in one breath, big change can be made. We know that bringing other like-minded individuals into our tribe makes our vortex bigger and more powerful, so there is support and unconditional love.

And it's as if no time has passed—as though we have been together all year long even though there are, in some cases, thousands of miles between us. I saw a friend of mine this last time and we both hugged for what seemed like hours, heart to heart. Then he looked me in the eye, said nothing and then looked at my daughters who are now ten and twelve. He said, "Dana, it's like I've watched them grow up. I've been witness to them becoming little women." There were tears in his eyes.

It's so true. You feel bonded with your tribe... over distance, time and life circumstance. You have definitely walked paths together before, and you can feel it the moment you embrace.

Your tribe holds space for you while you grow, while you stumble, and while you thrive. They hold space without judgment and without expectation. They do their thing in life and quietly applaud you while you do yours. There is unspoken gratitude for each other. The gratitude isn't about anything you have "done for them"; it's an appreciation for them living their passion because that gives you permission to live yours. You definitely are never off the hook in your tribe.

Your life could be similar or very, very different. It doesn't matter... because you only see one person. You recognize the oneness in it all. It doesn't matter where you've come from, what path you have walked, together or apart... there is only one.

The most potent thing a tribe does is remind you of who you are, where you came from, and why you are here. So when you leave that tribe, others who are not in your tribe or don't "get" your tribe, cannot vibrate in your field. Meaning that if you have been swayed in the past toward anything that is less than your highest light, you can no longer do that... comfortably. Your light grows stronger and more vibrant... it's as if you are fueled by the light of your tribe.

There is nothing more powerful than a tribe. If you haven't found yours yet, my advice is to stop, drop and look in the mirror. Don't look outside... look in your own heart.

One love... one heart... one tribe.

Upside Down

Handstand is about:

- Vulnerability... suspension between action and stillness.

- Sacrificing the illusion of safety or sure footing for illuminating clarity.

- Turning your perception upside down without expectation or attachment to the outcome.

- Forever shifting your perspective.

Handstand is inaccessible to many not because of lack of physical strength, but instead because of fear. It is unnatural to be upside down... or is it really?

Over the past year and half, my life has been completely turned upside down. To be honest, although the road was quite challenging, nothing in my life has felt more natural. Ironically, as I write this, it is the one-year anniversary of my magical trip to Tahoe, which marks the physical shift from my marriage to single life.

I remember last year in Tahoe very clearly. There was no way I could get into Handstand. I could not even consider Crow pose, to be honest. Basically, I couldn't perform one single pose on my hands. And believe me; it wasn't because I wasn't strong enough. It was fear—complete, deep, penetrating fear.

Where did this fear come from? Well, after many hours on my mat, on the phone with my mother, sitting in attorney offices across from my now ex-husband, and coddling crying children, I realize it was my deeply rooted beliefs that I could not support myself on many levels. It came from carrying so many responsibilities that to give up my life, as it was, for the freedom of the unknown, seemed absurd.

I was so afraid of loss... deep loss. Loss of respect, loss of my children, loss of financial security and friends. I was afraid of looking like a fool... both on my mat and off my mat.

I know this resonates with many people out there, because I have seen you, connected with you, talked with you and cried with you. I have listened to you while you too have had the carpet ripped out from beneath your "secure" lifestyle.

It is not easy to give up security and safety for the unknown. But isn't that faith? Isn't that listening to your heart? Isn't that really what every religion preaches... blind faith? And, funny... this is EXACTLY what it requires to shift your life or stand on your hands... blind faith. But oddly... when you do go upside down, or balance in ANY arm balance for that matter, you COMPLETELY shift your perspective. You shift your perspective on so many levels that, once you do this, you are forever changed.

This posture supposedly supports all the chakras through the heart chakra... of course it does.

Why? Because we HAVE to allow our hearts—not our heads—to lead us. Again, both on and off the mat. Fear is an illusion based on our mind creation. Love is not. I know what it is like to be afraid. I sat many an evening alone, sobbing uncontrollably, not knowing what to do next. I would wonder, *Where in the hell are all my friends? Why am I all alone in this?* But knowing beyond everything else there was infinite love and protection. That it had to be a journey I took alone. Just like Handstand... just like an arm balance... An instructor can't help you until you can support yourself.

And funny thing... This is truth... the day after I signed my divorce papers, I flew up into Crow and Handstand with ease and grace. Just did it... all on my own. A lot of this yoga stuff is a mind game, you know.

I'm telling you, you can do this. Listen to your heart. The ground will always be there. And when you choose to change the ground you walk on... all your faith will carry you until you find a new "home."

Who You Are

I purposely did not send out a blog for the New Year, welcoming you in. Why? Well, honestly, I knew you were doing your own thing and I was doing mine. However, now here we are in the New Year and I have to ask, how are you? Or should I say, who are you?

Our theme for this week has been "who are you?" Beneath the labels, the job titles, the busy-ness, the ambitious attitude, the resolutions, the sweat on your mat... who are you and what do you stand for? Because I've decided that's what really matters. The fire in your belly; the thing you would die for; the insane amount of love that overflows from you when you allow yourself to be vulnerable and trust.

It's crazy, really, once you decide to live like this. A bit chaotic at first but grounding does wonders.

You know this but I'll remind you: *Who you are is not the "likes" you get on your Facebook page, or how many Instagram followers you have, or even what people say about you in your testimonials on your site or to your face.*

I want to know who you are in the face of transformation. Who are you when you think your life is heading down one road and, all of a sudden, it takes a sharp left turn? Who are you in the face of adversity? Do you fall into fear? Do you stand alone and become the victim?

Who are you while you stand in prosperity and abundance? Do you honor your strengths and how you got there? Do you remember those individuals who lifted you up and held your hand? When you have more than enough, do you share?

I stepped into this New Year as strong as hell... ready to take on the world. Excited... elated... refreshed and clear about my path. Radiant, to be honest. Truth be told, my life is fantastic and I bow in gratitude every single morning before I ever leave my room. Because it wasn't always like this, and I know what a gift love is.

After four years of reorganizing, crying, doubting and struggling to remain in my space of light and love, I can finally say that I am "there." It feels amazing! I have my faith, my friends, my daughters and the light of the Goddess to thank.

Five days into the New Year I was knocked to my knees unexpectedly. Why? Because it was time for me to truly stand in my truth and really BE the pillar of strength that I am when I stand on my mat. You see, it's easy to stand in strength when we are "doing what we do." It's easy to BE that when it's an image to uphold or an idea to fulfill or even an example to set.

But at the end of the day, when the lights go out, or someone pulls the "wool over our eyes" and we are attacked to our core, that is when we truly see who we are, what we stand for and what we are made of. Do we forget the amazing magic and fall into the darkness? No, we keep moving... and moving into the light nonetheless.

We remember our infinite light and love and we keep moving in THAT direction. EVERY SINGLE THING that happens TO us happens for us. And we are ALWAYS being called to stand in a deeper integrity and truth of who we are with MORE grace and compassion than we can imagine we hold.

What do I stand for?

Truth. Integrity. Follow-through. Freedom. Justice. Love. Yes, all of that. And you know what? That hasn't changed about me since as far back as I can remember. And you what else? It's flippin' challenging to stand in that sometimes... especially when someone you have loved for so long takes that and challenges you to your core.

How do I handle it? With love, grace and understanding? Sure. I'll bow to it all with gratitude. And oh, by the way, I won't forget my sword that cuts through the bullshit with fierce compassion and authentic new boundaries.

We are always changing... always evolving and hopefully elevating ourselves to a level that represents a higher vibration of who we are in the light. And remember, the dark MUST ALWAYS be illuminated in order for the light to reflect its deepest essence... always.

Don't be afraid... go right into it. It's who you are beyond it all, IN it all. It's who you are.

Yogini Momma— The Great Balancing Act

As a mother of two young girls, I observe a lot, curse a lot, sleep in small doses and eat when I can. I love a good cup coffee and enjoy wine with friends. I do my best, and my kids will tell you that my best is far from perfect.

I like tie-dye pants and Lululemon gear. I scream at sporting events and chant at drumming circles. Given the choice, my girls would listen to MC Yogi rap about Ganesh over Justin Beiber any day. We operate as a team and there's no hiding anything. When we're upset, we say why and, to be honest, we argue a lot. They have their own minds and voices, and I try to listen up instead of talking over them.

But I have my doubts. I wonder if I'm doing it right, if I'm messing them up or if I made a huge mistake. I watch for negative patterns and breathe before I speak. I wonder if I am neglecting them at the expense of my career. I worry that I am neglecting myself while guiding their lives.

But here are a few rules that seem to work:

Respect each other's space.

> You know what's yours and what isn't; no games. Notice if someone needs love and just give it.

We are a team.

> When one is falling, pick up the slack. When one is rising, celebrate.

There is a time for play and a time for work.

> I will listen to every story about boys, pop-stars, books and movies, after your homework is done. You can have your phone back when you have a B+ in Math.

Everyone has a job, just do it without whining.

> No one is to blame but you when your job isn't complete. No pointing fingers.

Tell the truth, all the time.

> There is no excuse for lying. I might be upset or angry, but the truth always wins.

> *I ask them what they are afraid of, so I know. And I cuddle them at night. I will protect them with my sword and heart, but it is the letting go that's most important.*

I love my daughters something fierce. And I know many mommas who understand what I mean. The love we feel is deep, and we want to protect them from it all. At the same time, they must know how to protect themselves, live their passion, love others and function at a high vibration on this planet.

Our presence is what they want; it's how they thrive. But guess what? We can't give it to them every single second because we have to be present for other things too.

Break it down, be honest, be real and love them in as many fleeting moments as possible. At the same time, love yourself because that's the best lesson. They see right through the bullshit, they really do. Show them, lead by example, be there, but keep pulling away. They will love you later. Or so I'm told.

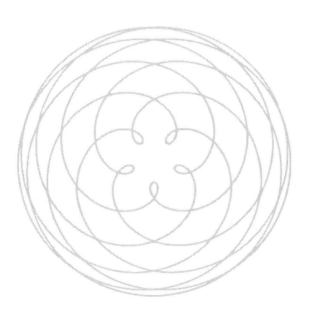

CHAPTER 2

Creative Passion
Svadhisthana Chakra

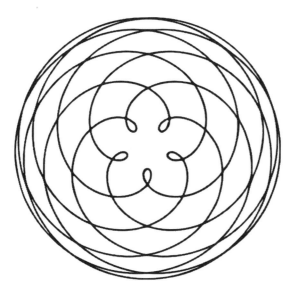

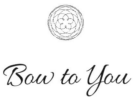

Bow to You

There are times in my life when I sit back and ponder. In fact, truth be told, I ponder a lot, maybe a bit excessively, but it has been so worth it. I call it a spiritual time-out. There is nothing like it... just sitting. Who DOES that?

Me. And apparently several other thousands of yogis on this planet. But sometimes we can all use a reminder.

I spent a weekend in Aspen a few summers ago, and I was again reminded how far we can come in just one year when we put our thoughts, words and actions into alignment.

I am not saying my life is perfect, far from it actually. But what is perfect anyway? Surely this moment is, especially when you sit back and remind yourself of all the events that brought you to it. There are no coincidences, only magical moments when the heart is open and flow happens.

This practice of yoga, of yoking your thoughts with your words and with your deeds, is a lifelong practice. It is a balancing act that takes effort, time and commitment. It is not something you wake up to and just do; you continue to BEcome.

The key to balancing it all is this: Take breaks. Get off the train of forward motion and ponder. Sit in grace. Sit in awe! Sit in complete presence and enjoy THIS moment.

Give yourself a huge high five for all the awesomeness you have created and how far you have come. Sit in gratitude for it all—every single bit—and see how each and every circumstance brought you to now.

When you do that you are sitting in the flow of life with a reverence that is light. You are sitting in a space that is open and vast. You are sitting in a space that is now, and it does not get any more real than that.

Make your plans, do your thing, BE your badass self, trailblaze, get it done. And then every now and again, sit in awe of yourself. Notice the greatness, the reflections, the tribe that surrounds you, the gifts and how much you have expanded.

Bow down... to you.

Empowered Grace

What does it mean to stand in empowered grace? Truth be told, I've been pondering, playing with and embodying this one all week long. And, I think we truly recognize what this phrase means when we are put into a position that requires the same amount of strength as it does poise, when we are being tested to stand in our truth and, not only that, but to speak it from a place of compassion and empathy.

Empowered grace comes into play when we are awake enough to whatever is happening that is causing discomfort and we can react in a way that exudes potency and breadth.

Here's an example. Visualize yourself being pushed into a corner... either physically, mentally, emotionally or spiritually. You know what I mean: those times when you are confronted and the primal emotion that bubbles up is fear, or anger or frustration.

The first thing you want to do is defend your honor, your stance, or your ego. Yeah, your ego. You've been side-lined so to speak, the wool has been pulled over your eyes, and all of a sudden you feel the urge to fight for something. You're not sure what. However, you feel the urge to defend something.

So you react without thinking. You allow your brain to fall into a patterned behavior. You add energy to the fear by becoming the fear and then the situation seemingly gets bigger and bigger. You allow this one situation to permeate your mind, pollute your heart, infiltrate your relationships and sabotage any type forward motion. Or, as I call it, a stalling of any up-leveled vibration.

At some point, after this same situation repeatedly happens, you decide it really isn't resonating with you any longer. And you're sure of it because you observe it all. You see how YOUR REACTION actually CREATES your reality and it just doesn't work for you anymore!

BINGO! YOUR REACTION creates YOUR REALITY.

It may take a few or several instances of the same event to resurface before you get it, but finally you do. And *this* time, this time you react with empowered grace. You sit silently and observe. You notice the pain, the anger, and the frustration bubbling up. You may even fall into fear for a moment. But this time, before it can escalate and permeate and poison anything else in your life, you breathe. You use a new tool... one that you've had all along, and you breathe.

You feel all the same emotions but you are empowered by them to do something different. You stand in them with your breath, a smile on your face, and you breathe. You notice how the emotion morphs and changes into perhaps grief or sorrow, and then you remember that whatever this is that's happening, it is a creation of your own mind and you know it's part of your evolution. And, all of a sudden, you are grateful.

WARNING: *You may feel empathy for the perpetrator, person or situation, and your heart may explode with compassion. This is a sure sign of evolution and a side effect of empowered grace.*

I always say... it's not if you do the pose, or even how you do the pose, it's how you fall out of the pose that matters. Yeah, that's empowered grace.

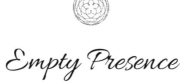

Empty Presence

"Empty presence can be said to be a mind without thought to clutter it; spaciousness, a sense of profound resting in non-doing."— Ariel Splisbury

Empty presence is moments when the mind is clear of thought and there is nothing but nothingness. And I say moments because when you realize you are in (or have achieved) empty presence, you have then dropped out of it.

It's a higher state of consciousness where you are open to receive, which goes against the very way we humans do things. The paradox of those moments is that in that nothingness, there is everything. You see, we have it all wrong. Our society would like us to believe that we have to do, prove, accumulate and achieve in order to BE, but that is not truth. Truth is being is just that... BE-ing.

Thankfully, we have this amazing mind that judges, categorizes and filters our thoughts daily. However, the mind is not the least bit concerned with the evolution of our soul. It is instead focused on survival, fitting in, and making things happen.

Did you know that we receive more information in a day than people received in their lifetime just 100 years ago? That's crazy! How can you possibly make any decision based on truth when you are getting pummeled—yes, pummeled—by stuff?

Everything you could ever want or need is a click away, and you better get yours! With this type of instant access to the Internet and social media, it's easy to fall into the old paradigm of "not-enoughness." Pssst... you are already enough...

This practice of empty presence is one that is important for anyone on the spiritual path. Why? Because you are no longer interested in surface skimming life. You are no longer involved in wallowing in everyone else's drama. You are no longer adamant in charging ahead to get what you want.

No, you are ready to dig deeper—into the sediment of your life. You are ready to use your power in difficult situations instead of giving it away. You are ready to syphon the sediment out and be completely clean and clear to receive whatever messages you are supposed to hear.

And, as I see it, with one click we are bombarded with everyone else's drama, ideas and beliefs. We give away our power left and right because we are subject to so much distraction that we couldn't possibly discern truth in a moment. We are so busy being busy that we don't have a moment to get to sediment, even though the sediment is what is driving every important decision in life.

Empty presence brings us to the stillness, the quiet, the spaciousness, and the vastness of all that is. It brings us to the nothingness that holds everything. It drops us out of our heads and into our hearts. It illuminates truth immediately.

And yes, it rustles up the sediment. The question remains, do you want to syphon it, or do you want to keep sitting on it?

In empty presence we are aware of our breath, we are aware of other's breath, we are aware of the consciousness that connects us, and we become aware that we are part of all that is. We fall into this amazing matrix of connection between us all. We see with our hearts and we realize that is all that matters.

- In empty presence we hear: We hear the call of our soul. We see ourselves as a part of the whole and experience that Oneness... for real.

- In empty presence we trust: We trust what we hear and we act on that trust and intuition, even when it goes against the ideas and concepts of others.

- In empty presence we know: We know that we are supported and that we can fly when we are ready; we know that we are held by the Universe and that it is safe to let go.

- In empty presence we receive: We receive all the grace, beauty and awareness that we will ever need in this moment.

Sit... sit with that for a moment. And then sit with it longer... especially if it's uncomfortable.

Freedom is a State of Mind

I have written about freedom several times now, and it's fun to look back and reread how I defined freedom on various occasions, along the timeline of my life.

I'm not surprised I like to write about freedom or that it evolves each time I come to it; I mean. the word is tattooed on my arm. Apparently, on some level it is important to me.

This time around I want to say this: *Freedom is a state of mind.*

How free you are can be directly related to how free your mind is from being sucked into the drama, circumstances, and issues of others. And believe me, this has been a hard one for me because, well, in the past I got sucked in pretty easily. But no more.

I stared at that moon last night, the night before, and many times before, honestly. I have stared at Her for many cycles and from many angles, asking Her about freedom. I have cried to Her in times when I felt like I was suffocating, compromising, losing, and dying. And She always, without fail, illuminated Her bright light, sharing her wisdom and grace with me.

As I look back on my past, which *is* in the past, I am inspired by own self. The path I have carved, the challenges I have overcome, the darkness I have owned, and the love I continue to share unconditionally.

- I bow to my teachers... the ones I love and the ones who I am challenged in loving.

- I bow to my embodiment of the word *empowerment* and how it has shown up over and over again.

- I bow to my new pattern of allowing love and support to come in, acknowledging it and offering it up, all in one swift breath.

I remember what it was like to not know if I would eat that day, where my next paycheck was coming from, or where I would be sleeping that night. I am grateful I can now watch my children ride their bikes to school, dance, sing and play sports when they want, and eat healthy food every day. I have felt the constriction of illusion and the expansion of truth. I have been in relationships that have sucked me dry and ones that have illuminated my heart so vastly I have felt deeply connected to the Divine.

Freedom is a state of mind that we can choose to experience in any given circumstance. We always have a choice to be free. Never once in those moments of perceived despair did I point the finger out or feel like I didn't have a choice. And if I did fall into that trap, you better believe some angel or teacher was there to remind me of something different.

That's what I'm doing for you now. In service of expansion and connection to the Divine.

I have been getting a lot of emails from self-proclaimed "healers" who offer to help you: "Free yourself from limiting beliefs and patterns that keep you stuck."

Free from negativity

Free from oppression

Free from drama

Free from disease

Free from stress and anxiety

Free from patterns

Stuck where, actually? Because if you are stuck somewhere, no one can get you out but you. No one can offer you freedom but yourself.

I looked outside myself for so long—so very, very long to find freedom. It was always there, in my heart, waiting to be recognized. It's there for you too. You just have to be willing to live in all that freedom... It's such a place of familiar calm you can't help but breathe into it and ask... Now what?

Gathering Energy

Eka Pada Rajokapotasana is all about re-gathering our energies and re-aligning with our purpose.

The world moves at warp speed; there is no denying that fact. With limitless amounts of information available at our fingertips, it's easy for even the balanced yogi to get overwhelmed and react. We can't help but be subject to emails, texts, Facebook messages and tweets. And, oh yeah, remember those face-to-face communications with people around us? Like your boss, your students, your partner, your children, yourself? Does that even happen anymore? And when it does, how authentic is the exchange? You certainly can't hit backspace, delete or rewind when talking with someone.

How grounded are you in your energy when you are communicating with someone one on one?

How connected are you to your own energy and what is going on in your body at any given time? Your cells? Your thoughts? How much of your daily actions come from a place of authenticity and how much come from a pure reactionary place? How connected are you to the repercussions of what you put in your mouth when you sit down for a meal? What about how much you allow the media... ALL MEDIA... to affect you and your energy?

You can't escape outside influence. You really can't... unless you go hide out on a mountaintop, I suppose. But you can find ways to insulate yourself and move through life with grace and strength.

Be advised here: Praying, meditating, doing yoga and chanting will NOT bring about perfection in your connections. However, I can promise you that with a compassionate practice, you CAN find more balance by setting that intention for yourself every single day. Not just Monday or Thursday, but every, single day.

The single-most important thing all of us can do, right now, is gather our energy and feel that security within ourselves, regardless of what is going on around us. It's been defined to me twice now as "being the eye of the storm." Being that pillar of clarity, stillness and serenity while everything else swirls around us, almost chaotically. Imagining a white light and violet flame surround us as life pummels us with curveballs, detours and lesson after lesson that we ourselves call in from a soul level.

It's truly our birthright to feel a sense of connection... to feel safe and at home within our own body, mind and soul. Feeling scattered or unsure of what your next step is, or when it is going to happen? If we can find that space, that magical space of breath, we can find our way "home" again.

Now, couple that with Eka Pada Rajokapotasana and you have yourself a winner! There's nothing like experiencing all your imbalances in Pigeon pose... the opportunities are endless! Name it... tightness in the neck, the shoulders, unevenness of the hips, tight hamstrings, ankles that hurt like hell in this pose. I often witness people clenching their fists in this pose... a sure sign of holding on tightly to some unconscious pain.

Our intention with this posture is to find our way home to breath. To relax into the posture, to feel the tightness and breathe into it with light and love. To melt and rehabilitate the joints, the muscles, the subtle body. To find balance and really make it a more natural part of our existence.

Remember it's just energy. It has got to move!

Just Three Simple Words

Just three simple words, that's all it takes to seed your life and set it into motion. But what happens is we are bombarded by so much more than three little words each day.

We veer off course because we allow our mind to go onto auto-pilot or over-drive listening to everything that's "out there." We co-mingle the beating of our own heart with the beating of another. We bump into other souls on their journey and ride along their path for a while, only to remember our own journey is what feeds our soul, not the path of another.

We are subject to more information in one day than people just over a century ago could even imagine. We can't possibly keep up with the whispers of our hearts!

Or can we?

Yes... yes, we can.

We stop and listen, and we listen often. We drop what we are doing and listen with our hearts, not our minds. We ask for a cue, a guide, a drop of nectar that fuels our movement forward and our ascension upward so we can be more of who we are in as many moments as possible.

So I ask you... with all that you have happening in your life in this moment, can you take a breath and drop into stillness? Can you sit for a moment, breathe and hear the whisper of your heart? What is it telling you? When you ask your heart, where can I expand, where can I grow, where can I open, what does it say?

Is there a situation in your life right now that requires your attention and care? Something that will offer you an opportunity to expand into a version of yourself that is more connected to Source and not just on auto-pilot patterns? What is one word that you can cultivate to do that? To be more aware, more present, more alive, more aligned with who you are?

When I look at my life, I see my heart... it's right there on my sleeve all the time. I look at my day-to-day and I am astounded by how quickly I manifest and how lovely this life is. I am always awestruck... always. And, when I manifest situations that, from the outside seem like a struggle, I remember the call of my heart. My heart called that in because it's just as beautiful as what I label as beautiful.

It, too, has the power to open up and expand in ways I can't imagine for myself. Those three words guide us and we have the opportunity to see them, experience them and embody them in every single situation.

What are your words? I've decided that while I have words for the year, I also am observing mine on a "moon-cycle" timeline now. So much happens in that time. I know one that is resonating so deep into my heart I feel like it will be here forever... beyond all time.

That's trust. Trust that all is working out in divine time. Trust that relationships will flourish into what they are meant to and that they may not be around forever. Trust in that, too. Trust that there is enough; trust that you are enough. Trust that Thy will is much more beautiful that your own will. Trust in the Universe.

That's my big word.

Others... **divine guidance, empowered grace, deep intimacy.** I know, it's more than three and there are adjectives before them. So I'm a bit dramatic sometimes... so what.

Find your words, write them down, experience them, embody them and then observe them showing up almost every single day.

Observe

The word *observe* fell into my lap last Sunday like a whoosh of energy. I never, ever plan out my theme for the week; it just comes. And this one was timely for sure. We had just experienced a full moon in Leo that shined a big, fat light on everything.

At the time, I observed all the amazing, creative, fiery energy that amplified EVERYTHING and KEPT ME MOVING FORWARD, even if I slowed down a bit to observe.

With Mercury in Retrograde still hanging out over everything that is good, just and expansive, there was this undeniable energy asking us to sit, slow down and observe.

Observe our emotions, our relationships, our opportunities and our patterns. This last week I swear I was watching a movie in slow motion called *My Life in HD*. I've had so many amazing things happen and, to be honest, I've had to look at some old, ugly stuff. Stuff that makes me so angry I could slap someone.

Yes, I do yoga, yes I meditate, yes I chant, and yes I eat healthy food. I keep my body, mind, and soul in a state of heightened awareness and pure consciousness to the best of my ability in as many moments as I can.

And I still want to flippin' slap someone. Well, just one person, truth be told.

And that is worth observing. Not so much that I let it consume me; just enough to change it—so I can change the paradigm for good. Yes, for good.

So while I have had this massive sinus cold all week, I've been cancelling appointments, staying in bed, sleeping, drinking everything green, still teaching classes and still tending to my children, I have been in a deep state of observation.

And you know what, I LOVE WHAT I SEE. I LOVE that I get to do what I do. I LOVE the people present in my life. I LOVE that I know how to say, "Help me please, I can't do this alone." I LOVE that I have these POWERFUL WOMEN in my life who propel me into being my best Self and expect nothing less. They cheer me on when I'm cursing about my issues and they give it to me straight so I stay in truth and the expansion of my OWN growth. I LOVE the men in my life who adorn me with affection, support and such masculine power I can't help but feel like a queen. And I LOVE that I get to hang out with my kids every morning and every night.

And...

I do not like my old reactions to being bullied, scared or hurt. I used to cower in the corner so as not to argue and keep the peace. I used to shy away from intimacy and vulnerability so as to look strong and invincible. And, I used to work so hard that I made no time for anything else but that. It's been a good time, hiding out. Staying safe, and out of the light just enough to not be that big, bold flame. Yes, it definitely served a purpose.

But it no longer serves me.

In this deep state of observation (somewhat forced; thanks Universe), I have truly seen my light. I have witnessed manifestation of prosperity, expansion, love and intimacy amidst what would have debilitated me a year ago.

Why? Because I have this amazing community of love and support showing up in my reality. And I've remembered, in this state of observing that it's just a reflection of... me.

So I ask you... what's showing up for you? What are you observing? What can you breathe into and expand? What discomfort can you sit in just long enough to evaluate, breathe into and shift your perception? When will you see the truth, which is that all your observations—every single one—are a reflection of an opportunity for you to evolve? Every, single one. I swear.

Passion

Foreplay started with that very first phone call. Ecstatic energy vibrated through the phone from your voice, penetrating my soul immediately. My heart skipped a beat and my breath became heavy. In my new life as a single woman, I had been enduring many a lonely evenings and this phone call was a welcomed variation.

"What's your biggest fear?" you asked me. "Being alone," I responded without thinking. "What excites you?" you inquired, "Life and a passionate existence." I had put my passions on hold for a few years and had forgotten what it felt like to be turned on by a voice—a sultry, sexy stranger on the other end of the phone. Truth be told, it had been awhile.

Before I turned my life upside down, I enjoyed an insatiable hunger for a deliberate, passionate existence. I loved life! Enjoyed it like it was a smorgasbord! Then life got real and I fell into survival mode. Your phone call rescued me; it was like putting the oxygen mask on.

I knew I had been with you before, in another life, potentially lifetimes over and over again. There was something so familiar, so safe, and so intimidating about you all at the same time. Just listening to your voice made my hands shake, my heart beat faster, and the hair on my arms stand on end.

When you suggested that we meet in person and that you come to visit me, I was thrilled and so very, very nervous. When I looked into your eyes, I knew our reunion was destined. I knew we had work to do. Our first meeting was powerful and when you pulled me to you, my loins were immediately warm and moist.

What was it? This connection... it wasn't like anything I had ever experienced before. I knew nothing about you, but everything was so familiar. The moment you touched my thigh, I heaved an exhalation that came from my soul. It was as if years of yearning were fulfilled with one touch.

Your hands on my body felt electric; they had roamed every inch of me before, and I couldn't get enough of you. Everything was magic, erotic, sensual and divine. It was as if time stood still from the moment you touched me, all the way to our epic climax.

Never once in all our meetings, our encounters, our intimate connections, did I know if I would ever see you again or where "this" was going. I never attached to any outcome, for no other reason than I never felt I had to.

However, in your absence I fell into humanity; overridden by my ego and overcome with fear, I drew a line in the sand because I had to. You triggered me like no one else ever had. You pulled away for no reason, and then pierced my heart with thoughtless words. At the time, I didn't have the tools to hear what you were really trying to say; I defended my territory instead of trying to understand.

Our arguments were swift, fierce and familiar. I had never suffered that type of irrational outburst, but I knew they were uncovering a recurring old story told by my heart revealing deep pain, grief and disappointment.

It became easier to keep you at arms' reach where I could control how deeply I let you in. And when you got too close, emotionally penetrating my heart, reopening wounds, I told you to leave. Not because I didn't love you deeply but because I was afraid of what that love would excavate from my past. I was afraid of how lovely the light would be and how brightly it would shine in my life.

When you left for the last time, I endured; in fact, my life flowed effortlessly. It was much easier to be busy, to keep my life moving at a backbreaking pace, actually, so I could avoid the grief. That deep passion had disappeared, never to be replaced by anything even close to what we shared. My heart hurt and my body ached for you. It was if I was missing a limb. I woke up many nights, sweating, crying and more than once I was awakened by the most powerful orgasm.

Now I knew what "You're in my soul" meant. You definitely set up shop in my soul.

To move forward, I transformed that intimate passion into my life-affirming passion. I used it to fuel my own life in a way I may not have been able to do had you not shown up. Our meeting gave me the courage to look inside and realize that I possessed that passion for life in my own heart, without the need for outside recognition, acceptance or acknowledgment.

Would I have found that without our exchange? Sure. Were you an amazing catalyst? Absolutely.

When I saw you again, this last time, compassion, forgiveness and unconditional love expanded in my heart. I softened and opened up to love, completely. Your touch, your lips, your skin, though weathered and obviously older, still excited me beyond explanation. The moment you touched me, my heart rate escalated and my breath became heavy.

Beyond time and distance, regardless of our past or other lovers, our relationship remained the same. Through this unexplainable connection and deep unconditional love, I learned to enjoy this moment, because this moment is all we can ever count on.

Passion is underrated; it's replaced too often by obligations, responsibilities and stagnation. It's pushed to the side in exchange for a perception of safety. Let me say this: Safety is an illusion; passion is real.

It's also seen as something that we find outside of ourselves. I believe that sometimes, as spiritual beings living a human experience, we forget that we have the ability to experience a passion for this life all on our own.

And sometimes we need that erotic, primal, animalistic instinct to push us forward.

Maybe that's just me... maybe I'm the only one who actually enjoys dropping the illusion of control every now and again, if only for a moment, for an intimate exchange of ecstatic bliss. But I doubt it.

I have had the privilege to experience a complacent life, disillusioned by what I would have called mundane, unable to find passion in anything at all. And I have tasted that primal knowing of ecstatic bliss in one moment, in one breath and in a heated exchange of love and intimate connection.

A connection beyond explanation, beyond reasoning, and resting only in an intuitive ignition of two souls coming together in union.

Personally, I would rather experience that primal force of Shakti, even the potential of it, if only for a moment, with no promise of ever feeling it again, than a lifetime of mediocre companionship. Why? Because I am already all that I need, and if I experience that bliss if but once, I am blessed beyond belief. Because that force that is beyond explanation, beyond reason and beyond anything that makes sense is the fire that sparks life itself; it's the fire that lifts the veil of our own illusions and reminds us just how powerful we are.

Shaktis-Call-to-Shiva

I send this out to all beings who are ready for partnership. Not because they need it or they are not whole without it, but because they know, deep in their bones that when they thrive, the planet thrives. They know that it is the way of the Divine Feminine and Sacred Masculine: to BE in partnership. They understand that the way of a patriarchal society is over and we are calling our partners home.

Know that in this readiness, there isn't a need for partnership. The joining together actually brings more aliveness, motivation and support to both parties.

Energetic connection is what fuels these divine souls. Connection goes without saying and devotion is unspoken. However, physical connection and a warm embrace satisfies the human existence and brings comfort and support to a restless heart and spirit.

He is strong and courageous and is there for me in all my humanity. He isn't just physically holding me, he is big enough and **strong enough to hold my emotions, my fears and my worries**. So much so that they dissolve into his masculinity. I am fueled by his presence alone, for that is what I need to continue my work on the planet as a Goddess, a mother, and a truth-seeking spiritual warrior: the presence of the Masculine.

Because of this energetic support, I am free to do my work in the world and am able to support and love him for his Godlike presence. For he has work to do as well and needs the support of the Goddess.

I am available to shower him with love, affection, intimacy and sexual connection beyond his wildest dreams because that is what he needs to be the man he desires to be in the world. **Adoration, gratitude, and a deep bowing to his greatness.**

When we come together, there is not you and me, there is only "us." He loves my children immensely but doesn't try to replace their father. Instead, he shows them what it means to be a man in the way he treats me as his partner and them as little Goddesses. He has no problem supporting me in my parenting if I ask, but shows up in support of me, and that is enough.

We enjoy working together because we share the same passions and know it's time to put them out into the world together. We do have work that takes us away from each other, but we are fueled by the separation. **We are as comfortable in the space between us as we are in the connection when we are together.**

Our sexual connection is magic and divine; when we converge in this way, time stands still and our breath becomes one. **He knows just how to light my internal fire and can excite me just by breathing in my presence. An orgasm is a powerful way to ignite Shakti and creativity,** and when I am being fed in this way, my work and connection with everything outside of that thrives. It is essential to this powerful Goddess. Essential. There is enough-ness in cuddling and spooning, to be sure, but there is nothing like a man who can stimulate this Goddess incarnation.

My masculine partner must be able to stand up to me. NO PUSHOVERS, please. NO YES MAN, thank you. He must desire and partake in open, authentic, supportive communication that is beneficial to the growth of both parties.

We both allow space for each other to shift and grow and provide support in that shift, comfortable or not. This makes our bond special and divine.

Our egos get the best of us at times, and when that happens each of us hold space for the other's moment of hesitation, drop into what is real and then move into expansion. **We will come back to the heart where only love resides and BE that for each other.** We know arguments, miscommunications and misunderstandings happen in times of growth, so we both support these instances with grace, compassion and love.

My man has claimed me and is not afraid to say it. Everyone knows how much he adores me because he isn't shy about admitting it. Public displays of affection are necessary and a part of our existence. He is excited to see me and be with me. He knows that I am special. He bows to my existence and adorns me with love, grace, presence, and romantic times together. He is an exceptional role model of what it means to be a man. My daughters witness this, changing their paradigm of what a loving relationship looks like and feels like.

We spend time in nature, traveling the globe, relaxing at home and in love together or apart. There is a definite balance of learning, loving, growing and supporting of each other. Each of us has something of importance to offer, and our connection never gets old or stagnant.

He knows that I am a strong warrior Goddess and can hold space for the little boy that still lives inside of him. He can be himself in authenticity and vulnerability. **He isn't afraid of dissolving his ego over and over and can find ways to work through his stuff with and without me.** I am a container that holds infinite space and he uses it wisely. He knows he can be himself in all forms and that I have the capacity to love it all as one.

In return, he sees all of me. He is witness to all the dynamics and intensities of my soul: *the Goddess, the warrior, the Momma, the entrepreneur, the space holder, the woman, the little girl...* he navigates them all with grace and ease.

He is confident and knows that once I have committed I will never leave. I have attracted my sacred masculine and I am devoted to that connection and intimacy. He is special and so am I. He is conscious and so am I.

We love love, sex, travel, intimacy and this planet.

We are ready to receive each other in grace, gratitude, strength and potency. We have done the work and know that every experience has led us here... to each other. We am perfectly imperfect and worthy of such musings. I am an evolved woman and he is an evolved man. **We have been waiting for each other and we will not settle for anything less until we finally gaze into each other's eyes, knowing that it is time. That we have found each other.**

It is done, it is done, it is done... and so it is.

Truth

Wow... wanna know the truth? This Mercury retrograde and full moon in Sagittarius is kicking my ass! I've been tossed into amazing opportunities and yanked back into the past all in one week. I had to face my immobilizing fear of technology and fix every i-apparatus in my home, by myself. I have to buy a new computer, and I lost all my photos of my children from 2002 (yes, I heard that gasp).

I found the photos but I had to ask my wusband for a copy of them on disk and dig into my dusty storage unit to find the printed copies. This was before my meeting with Dove, after I sent in my grant proposal to Lululemon, and while I was training two new amazing yogini-support goddesses and booking three events for Girls Elevate™. Oh, and of course there's the lovely mini-goddesses who had signing recitals, band concerts, math issues, drama issues, boy issues, and are gearing up for summer like middle-school kids do.

I feel like I'm hitting it all out of the park! Well, maybe a few times I've had to stop at first or second base, but at least I'm hitting it and not striking out. And those stops were potent, powerful, and very necessary. Because that's what I used to do, not even try, pretend to be sick or ill-equipped, or skip to home plate without touching a foot on first, second or third.

I would hide my truth behind perfection. I was living in a world that was riddled in a perceived sense of safety and stability. And you know what that felt like? Prison.

I have TRUTH—FREEDOM—LOVE tattooed on my arm. I got that tattoo exactly one year after I divorced and exactly two days before I picked up my life and moved to California. Yes, the truth is, it's taken this long to get to that place of pure acceptance—a place that holds no resentment, anger, or frustration. And, quite possibly, why I need one more year to complete it.

Here is what I have learned about truth.

It's not just about telling the truth, it's about knowing the truth. You can't possibly know your truth when you're wrapped up in everyone else's drama. It's just not possible.

It's not about speaking your truth, it's about living it and owning it. And just in case you aren't aware, the truth isn't always pretty. Nope... it can be wrapped up in addiction, fear, guilt and resentment.

It's not just about knowing your truth; it's about feeling it from the inside out. Truth isn't some superficial, cordial, obligatory post on Facebook. Truth is felt in your gut, and it spills out of you silently sometimes because it just needs to be acknowledged by you and you alone.

Oh, and it's not just about living it and owning it either, it's about sharing it from a place of humility that heals others and yourself in the process. This is why I love yoga and why I'm fully vested in Girls Elevate, along with raising my two daughters consciously.

Because you see, in my past there was abuse, and drugs, and too much unconscious sex and not enough empowerment. Because there was fear, guilt, and shame. I'm not the only one experiencing this wake-up call either; I witness many of you with the same story as my own. This isn't a pity party; this is a coming out party.

Here's what I say: enough of the blame, the pointing fingers, the untruths and foolishness. None of that matters. Not one single bit.

Own your truth and know that it is ever evolving. You know what that means?

That your truth now, in this moment, is most likely different from the truth of, say, your adolescent self. I know mine is. But the question is, how long do you hold onto that old truth and live it as your now? Using it as an excuse not to shine your light or God forbid, perhaps help others find theirs.

I'll repeat what my teacher Sean Corne said to me (and to a class of about 100 others) in 2009 that shook me to my core: *"How dare you live a life that is mediocre. How dare you know how beautiful you are and not share that gift? How dare you use any excuse to not live your dream? How dare you?"*

Your truth... your light... your gift... is sitting there, wanting to be metabolized into manifest form—meaning it wants to be birthed in this life. It's your job to own it!

If you're watering it down in fear, not listening to it because you can't hear it, not expressing it because you are afraid to fail, the time is now to stop doing that and get on the ledge and live it.

I know it's scary, but my credo is better to have tried and failed than to never have tried at all. Do not live a life of regret or of not trying. And you want to know what? I'm ready to live an up-leveled version of my truth. Because there's no place to go but up, all the time... to infinity and beyond!

The cool thing is your truth is always evolving, always. So whatever you are experiencing now can be lived or changed. And the absolute best thing about it is, you get to drive.

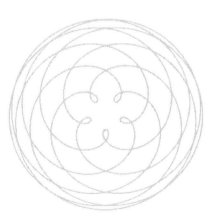

CHAPTER 3

Power and Transformation
Manipura Chakra

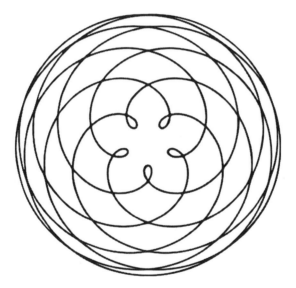

Celebration

In November 2012, I left Vancouver, Washington in a hurry. Like ripping a Band-Aid off, quick, without thinking, cringing from the pain, and hoping the air would heal my wounds.

I wasn't running away and I wasn't trying to hide. I just had to get out from underneath the bazillion labels I had created for myself in the nine years I had lived there. They were no longer serving me and I just could not do it while continuing to live there... I wasn't strong enough.

Moving away and starting over wasn't easy—not even in the least bit—but that's another story. This one is about celebration.

Seemingly, there wasn't anything to celebrate at the time. In my selfish haste, I pissed a lot of people off, I disappointed even more, and perplexed even myself. You see, I put myself in a position where I had no one to rely on but myself. And during that time I faced every single fear I ever had from as far back as I can remember. And I did it all alone—which was indeed one of my fears.

What's to celebrate?

- Coming out on the other side witnessing friends expose their heart with unconditional love and acceptance.

- A strong, sturdy warrior who exudes love, compassion, gratitude, strength and wisdom.

- Relationships that were challenging, triggering and tough as nails, now healed and full of grace and mutual appreciation.

- A community of people alive, ready and excited about waking up to who they are.

- Insight to truth... real truth.

- Embodiment of spiritual connection and authenticity that has been portrayed on the mat, now flowing off the mat... for real.

- An appreciation for my entire life and for every single person who has crossed my path and taught me something.

You see, I think sometimes when we are living in our day-to-day, we forget about how magical life is. We forget that we have the power within us to heal, to forgive and to love. We forget that we can live a life that is magical in just about every moment. We forget that everything is for our higher purpose, our soul's evolution.

So... What do you have to celebrate?

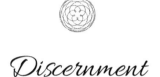

Discernment

How can we possibly discern what is true for us and beneficial for the evolution of our soul when we are bombarded by life? And by *bombarded* I don't mean that we've lost control some how. I just mean, sometimes life moves at the speed of light and, honestly, we start to move at that speed without knowing it and that's not always the best thing.

Discernment is defined as *the ability to judge well*. What does that mean, anyway? To judge well? I'm not sure I agree with that definition. In my humble opinion, discernment can be best described as:

> *A moment in time where we are offered an opportunity to know what is right for us. A moment in time when we choose what resonates deep within our heart. A moment in time when we make a choice that best suits the evolution of our soul.*

I like to think of it as the space between breath and reaction. The quiet stillness between the conflict of the ego and the soul. An internal knowing of what is elevating us and what is contracting us. It's the emotional time-out we take before reacting from a patterned, triggered place.

The issues with discernment, as I see it, are instant gratification and old triggers.

We have this appendage we call our phone, and it can get us the information we need right when we need it. The question is, do we really need it? And do we really need it in that moment? If we can find what we think we need, in a moment when we think we need it, are we offering up space to evaluate if we really even need it or not?

Maybe not. Then we're left with information taking up brain space that we really didn't need.

Old triggers... yeah, you know what I'm talking about. Something happens that is not really in alignment with your "chi" and you fly off the handle. You say something that feels "old," react in a way that is less than love and then you're left standing there wondering "who the hell was that person?"

How to remedy this? You take a breath. FYI, it's free. And it feels good.

In that one breath, space is infinite, presence is palpable, love is emanating, and the soul is ignited. In that moment, that one moment in breath, we are offered a second to discern what is really happening. And we are better able to act from a place more in alignment with our soul.

Discerning what is real, not judging what is right. This one simple act can change the world.

Discipline

Discipline is defined as *a branch of knowledge or the practice of training people.* I find this interesting as a yoga "teacher," for a few reasons. One is that that while I am a teacher, I am also only a student. And honestly, the only person I am ever really training is myself.

I mean, sure, I lead classes, workshops, and trainings; facilitate retreats; and sincerely enjoy mentoring and coaching people. However, at the end of the day, I am actually up leveling my own knowledge and devotion to this practice. Not only that, but I'm constantly learning about relationships, spirituality, connection, and business just with my "work." And this is because everything I am experiencing is a reflection of me. Every person I am privileged to meet and discover has something to share with me.

Remembering this simple fact, by the way, takes a TON of discipline.

And, to be completely transparent, the real discipline for me is what I do with all that stuff I say and share on my mat. With discipline, I take it off my mat and into my own, real world—the one that is riddled with adolescent girls, tasks that never end, creation and connection, and a new commitment to daily self-care and empowerment.

So I feel like the word *discipline* could almost be synonymous with commitment, but with complete awareness. Meaning that if we really looked at our life and what we "want," we have to ask ourselves, are we disciplined enough to not be distracted by every ding, ring-tone, notification, and message we receive that is not on our path of teaching/learning? Can we really discern that for ourselves? And, if so, how long does it take?

> I use the word like this: *I am disciplined in my practice. I am disciplined in my thoughts. I am disciplined in my desires.*

More than anything, though, I think it is vitally important to discipline our breath. And that is the simplicity, the sacredness, the ease and practice of yoga.

Here's the deal: If you can discipline your breath—meaning teach yourself to focus only on a rhythmic cadence of your breath—you can begin the practice of creating your life in just the way you desire.

How?

Well, when you discipline the breath, you take a moment to focus on nothing but the breath. And in that nothingness, there are countless thoughts. And you, in that one breath, are offered the opportunity to "stick with it" or "distract." And what's so very important about this is that we are fed so much information in a second, in an hour, in a day... that we can't possibly keep up with it all. Not only that, but we really don't even need it all.

And in that one breath that we take, very consciously, we are offered a nano-second to discipline our thoughts so they are more in alignment with who we are and what we desire. We can notice before we react; before we fall into a pattern; before we go down the "wrong" path.

So, when I begin sharing this practice or this discipline, I like to ask:

How serious are you about your practice? What are your intentions? Are you disciplined enough to stay focused? To the end? To find the joy in learning, falling, growing?

Because this discipline, this practice, this journey of yoga is not for the faint of heart. It is for those individuals ready to wake up to it all. And, mostly when it gets difficult, they are the ones that sit in a pose that is uncomfortable, breathing into the tight spaces of their body so when they experience that constriction off their mat, say in relationship, they can breathe into that, too, with the same grace, awareness and acceptance.

To me, that is discipline.

Fierce Action

You know, I have been sitting—sitting for quite some time. Sitting in my stories, sharing them as a way to heal and inspire. Sitting in my breath, hoping it will smooth over the rough edges of my past so I can fully move forward. Sitting in silence so I can hear the voices from my heart over all the noise. Sitting and chanting to Ganesha, Lakshmi, Krishna, Shivya... to anyone who will listen.

I've chanted *Om Gan Ganapataye Namah* and *Om Namah Shivaya* until my throat was raw.

I have been sitting so long my ass hurts.

I'm done sitting. I'm not saying I'm done meditating, chanting, learning, believing, affirming, sharing, or healing. No, quite the contrary; all that was my beacon through rough times; it brought me to now. As I continue to fumble through mantras, deities, asana and hearing my own voice, I know I am a life-long student. I am however, acknowledging a shift—a shift to deeper integration.

The difference is I AM all THAT while I am moving through my life. Because I'm ready to move. I feel the push of the moon and the Universe; I hear the call of God and it is time.

It is time for clear, concise, fierce action. I've had so much brewing inside and it has needed time to formulate or percolate, if you will. It has needed time to sweep cobwebs away, to focus in, to dial in the aperture, so the path would illuminate so brightly that there was no question, no hesitation. Whichever way you want to metaphorically phrase it... it is clear and it is time.

This idea of Girls Elevate came to me years ago and I'm finally now, after all this sitting, ready to bust it out.

It's time.

The sitting is as important as the movement... it's the balance of the Shiva and the Shakti. Sitting has to happen... but then movement must follow. As we mosey along our path, each step is important. Just because "it's time" doesn't mean it's time for the Grand Finale or the Great Spectacular. "It's time" could mean it's time to evaluate, or collect, or clean up, or clean out, so that when you do move, you move in a way that is swift and conscious like a deer.

Yeah, that's where I'm at today... swift and conscious like a deer. What are you ready to bring into manifestation? What have you been sitting on for awhile now? Do it. The Universe has your back.

Leaping Forward

A grasshopper leaps only forward... it never leaps backward! When you think about it, that really makes so much sense.

Leaping forward for us humans means trusting your instincts, joy, abundance and virtue. It means living from your heart and not your mind. It means trusting your gut and not overanalyzing every detail that you most likely don't have control over, anyway. It means saying yes before you know every single, potential consequence of your choice.

Let me ask you... how often do you do that? REALLY trust your instincts? REALLY live from your heart? Say yes without examining what might happen?

Too often, our own minds hold us back; we get in our own way. We stay in unpleasant situations far too long because we are afraid of any myriad of things: being judged, getting hurt, making the wrong decision, failing. So we stay stagnant... only to find that the same opportunity to leap shows up again in a different form.

Leaving the familiar behind isn't always easy. Especially if it involves a jump of some kind. But, if we truly take on a practice of trust in EVERY-THING—our own power, divine guidance, universal influence and love—taking a leap becomes natural. Just like a grasshopper.

I have never regretted any leap I have taken—not ever. Leaps give us perspective, strength and grace.

While you are leaping you are learning. When and if you fall, you are learning. What you witness along the journey, you are integrating. And the other side of the leap offers perspective, wisdom, insight, and most often, compassion.

So take the leap; what's the worst that can happen? Really?

Before I leap, I always ask myself which is worse: staying stagnant, not saying how I really feel, being caught up in complacency; or falling on my face in the name of vulnerability and truth? I have fallen on my face many times, but every single time it has been so worth it!

Navigating Change

With this season's change, I am again reminded of the law of impermanence. Nothing stays the same. Nothing. As I watch the leaves turn, feel the winds blow and sense the change in the air, I quickly remember that we are no different than the trees. We too, yearn to flow with nature and its faith in what is.

The summer of 2013 was when this lesson was more palpable than ever before! It was the summer I moved my children from the Pacific Northwest to live with me in Northern California. And while my ex-husband and I both knew that theoretically, it was for the best, it still sidelines us all every now and again.

All summer we played, hiked, met new people and enjoyed each other. Being the momma bear that I am, I strived to make things as "normal" as possible for them. But the reality was that it wasn't normal; the minute they stepped foot on California soil, everything changed. Some days that change is like a gentle breeze that blows through our life. And on other days it's like a flippin' tsunami and we are all pummeled to the ground.

As I watched them navigate new friends, new schedules, new sports teams, new EVERYTHING, I was both proud and inspired by them. Their openness; their trust in me and in their dad; their strength, honesty and trust in this Universe. But even the bravest of souls cry out when things get a bit like a dust storm.

It's change—transformation—newness. Some of us thrive in it and some of us hunker down, clinging to what was because it's familiar and feels comfortable. But the reality is that nothing is permanent. Now to be fair, transformation and change, letting go, doesn't have to be a radical event. You can let go of something small… you can change your life two degrees and create a brand new path for yourself.

I guess the depth of your change depends on just how much you have accumulated and how much you cling to stuff, people and ideas.

So how do you navigate through change and letting go, especially when it involves other people?

1. Just sit with it all. Sit in the uncomfortablness. Sit in the grief, the pain, the fear… feel all of it. Just be with it all because it will move through you. Don't try to fix anything and don't try to stuff it down.

2. Look outside your box of life and see what's waiting for you to embrace, to love, to cherish and to be grateful for. Sometimes we cling so desperately to what we thought was ours, we miss out on what's sitting there, just waiting to be recognized.

3. Look for the lesson. And there is one… for your growth and evolution.

4. Subscribe to the belief that there is enough—enough money, enough time, enough love, enough of everything—and when you let go, more will come. It's a law.

5. Let go gracefully, with love, gratitude and compassion for what was (even if it hurts) and what is. And then be open to the miracle of what comes next.

6. Have trust… trust that the Universe is handing you everything you need, because if your hands are full you can't receive, right?

After your tantrum of wanting something and not getting it, wishing circumstances were different or trying to change things to your liking, and after the tears have subsided, take a breath and look around you. Be with what is… be in your stuff and you will witness such beauty and grace it will astound you.

Without guilt, shame or worry… just be and know that the navigation is bringing you to a higher version of yourself.

On the Other Side

Wow... was that a shakedown or what? I mean, REALLY? Did anyone else feel that to their core? This last month was exactly as predicted, with some unexpected twists and turns. When the Universe starts aligning like that, it's almost as if there is an audible roar that comes from the depths of the Earth, and we all feel it.

Talk about shifting, releasing, realigning, calling in truth, moving into your purpose; yeah, it's been all that! AND the solar eclipse with the New Moon has yet to grace us on Wednesday!

Seemingly, the aperture of my life dialed into such clarity, it was almost blinding at times. I kept trying to look away but I just couldn't. Everything magnified and became so large and so clear it was impossible not to see truth.

This new moon is meant to bring refinement to all this shifting, which is a relief. As I accept this overwhelming clarity, I'm still experiencing uncomfortable tremors. Personally, I would feel much more relaxed with a hum instead.

I witnessed shifts in every area of my life... and, thankfully, they weren't epic tsunamis this time. No, this time the shift was just enough to upgrade relationships, revise my career path, expand my intuitive capabilities, improve my health, and wake me up, just that much more.

The difference is gratitude. Because, as we shift, there is a pause... a pause in the breath so that we make space for seeing the grace in it all.

When we breathe gratitude in and out, we rest, we listen, we sleep soundly, we watch, we allow. We don't *do*, we just are. Personally, I purified, I prayed, I snuggled, I let go, I felt into it all with gratitude for every emotion. And now...

I accept only authenticity and truth 100 percent of the time. I've fallen into the eyes of love. I know my worth and what I deserve, and I accept nothing less than greatness. I know my purpose and step into it eagerly. I see above the haze and no longer spend any time there.

Life is too short to play small... to settle for less... to be afraid of your light. Every morning is a brand new opportunity to BE you. Guess what? In all that transition, a lot of your stories that held you back got left in the rubble. You can spend time looking for them and reliving them or you can move forward into the light you came here to be. What's it gonna be? Because it's a new day and you get to decide.

Onward and Upward

Seems to me that there is a whole lot of shifting happening these days. And at the same time, seemingly these shifts and events are synchronistically working as we watch in awe.

I can't even begin to count the number of conversations I have had in just the last month that have ended in, "Of course I was supposed to meet you!" or "Wow, I can't believe I ran into you HERE, of all places!" or "I was JUST thinking about you!" or "Hmm... isn't that interesting how these events have brought us together?"

Do you believe in coincidence? I don't. I think that everything happens in divine order, actually. I also believe that right now, on this planet, at this time, the Universe is TOTALLY conspiring to bring all the light seekers, way showers, shift makers and leaders together because it is time to make a difference.

It is really important to note that these people to whom I am referring aren't coming to me in this space of blissful happiness, yellow light shooting from the crowns of their heads. No, it is more like they are showing up almost like... well... like they just fell out of their washing machine after a massive spin cycle. Like a hurricane just came through, blew through their life and rearranged everything.

They are experiencing change, turmoil, loss and profound, deep lessons that have shown up as a recurring event that they can't seem to shake. What's beautiful to note is that because they are awake, they are observing and noticing the patterns. Maybe this is you... maybe not.

Regardless, what I can say is this... notice. Wake up and notice what is happening in your life. First off, it is ALWAYS a reflection of your thoughts. Second, it is ALWAYS an opportunity to move forward.

Ask yourself this when you wake up from your slumber:

> *How do I want to show up now in my life? What do I envision now that I am alive and moving forward? What does my life look like with regard to relationship, career, finances, environment and spirituality?*

We are consistently offered opportunities to grow, to change and to elevate. The wonderful thing is that we get to choose the path, the rate of speed and the height of growth. That's right, WE choose. We can slow it down; we can speed it up; we can sit in it; or we can move past it.

So when you SEE, really SEE the change happening, when you notice the opportunity... what are you going to do? Will you continue to sit in the lesson, analyzing and picking it apart for more clarity? Will you continue to wait for the "right time" to move forward with a plan, idea or relationship? Will you continue to allow love and light to pass you by while you try to understand it all?

Or will you sit with it all, just long enough to feel compassion, gratitude, love and peace with it. JUST LONG ENOUGH to feel it and honor that change for what it represents, which is growth and elevation of your soul.

It is time to pinpoint that which you really are and embody it. Sit with your stuff just long enough to bless it and move forward. There really is no other way.

Power

I love this word, *power*. Powerful, powerless, powering through, empowered... it's so versatile and strong and, well, powerful.

As always, I looked up power and one definition was: *the capacity or ability to influence the behavior of others or direct the course of events.*

This definition resonated big time. And it got me thinking a lot about the way we humans use our power. Because the truth is that we all hold such great, great power...

But the question is how do we use it?

I've seen it used so many ways: Empowerment of others. Advancement of an idea. Transformation of a situation. Influencing the growth of an individual as well as a community. I've also seen power used to instill fear and create guilt. I've witnessed people using their power to get what they want without any regard for anyone else. And I've seen power being abused in many inequitable relationships.

And this type of behavior isn't just employed in big corporations or political offices; no, this type of behavior is exemplified in yoga communities, small companies, school yards, on the Internet, in relationships, and behind closed doors.

The truth is, **the reason behind every single disagreement in every single relationship is an imbalance of power**. Power over another can ruin and rule a lot of our relationships.

I mean, we are very powerful beings, flinging our power all over the place, in any one given moment. Are we conscious when we use this God-given power? Are we using it for the benefit of all individuals involved?

Best to know what you want and then discern whether that desire for power is coming from a conscious place or an egoic need. Making the wrong decision could mean cleaning up lots of karma later.

Are we consciously utilizing our power in a way that is compassionate, admirable, and yet beneficial? And is it in balance with just how much power we are allowing others to express?

> *Power over money, power over decisions, power over sex, power of earning capability, power over the community, power to make the final choice.*

On the flip side of expressing our power is examining how often and how easily we give our power away. Because that is such an easy thing to do, without even knowing we're doing it.

> *Saying yes when you mean no. Avoiding confrontation to keep the peace. Allowing someone to speak on your behalf. Not standing up for what you believe in just because you're afraid of something that is probably irrational anyway.*

I hear people say, "he took my power away" or "she wouldn't let me be myself" or "he made me feel this way." And now, this whole bullying thing that has become an epidemic in our schools, at work, and on the Internet has gotten me thinking about power.

The truth is this:

> *You were born with power and you are in charge. Period.*

> *You are the one who has to learn how to use it in a kind, beneficial way.*

> *And no one—I mean no one—can take it away. Ever.*

We willingly give our power away and we manage just how we use it. Period.

I know some of you out there are saying, "Oh really? What about war? What about rape? What about divorce? What about adultery? What about terrorism? What about sex trafficking? What about these horrific things that go on every day that some of us in our bubble don't even pay attention to?"

I get it. It hurts my heart; some of these things that are happening around the globe that we have absolutely no control over. And we sometimes feel powerless to do anything.

I get it.

But here's the deal... We can manage ourselves and only ourselves. We can choose how we use our internal power to make things right, to ignore, or to pray. We can stand up for what we believe is true and right and just, and we can pray that our efforts create something different.

I tell my girls, all the time: No one can make you do anything, ever. Not even me. I can only suggest, challenge and redirect. At some point they have to make their own decisions on how best to use their power.

And that of course, led me to the idea that if this were indeed true, you can never be a victim. And that in actuality, every single time that you have felt powerless, you have given it away. Unconsciously or consciously.

When you recognize that you have complete responsibility and jurisdiction over your power, life takes on a whole new meaning.

Why?

Because if you gave it away, you can get it back. Anytime you want.

You can get it back.

And that is power.

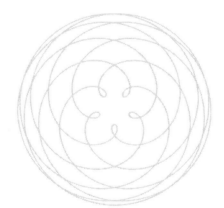

Quakes and Ripples

I was pretty shaken up by the earthquake that hit at 3:20 a.m. Sunday morning. I hadn't felt that much shaking in years and the energy was violent. I went from sleeping to bolting to my daughters' room while still sleeping... kind of like you do when you hear your newborn cry: instinctual, protective movements.

My heart was beating out of my chest when I walked into their room as I witnessed my older one sitting up, frozen with wide eyes. She said, "Momma what is that?" Calmly, heart on my chest, I said, "It was a little earthquake honey, but it's okay now. You can go back to sleep." To which she replied, "Will it happen again?" And I, of course said, "No honey, you can sleep now."

I went back to bed once I knew she was sleeping, but there was no way I was going to fall asleep. I grabbed my phone to read what had happened. Fifteen texts had come through. We were all feeling it.

A meditation seemed appropriate but I couldn't get myself out of my bed again. Tears rolled down my eyes as I dove deep into my heart, out of fear and into love. I lay there praying to all the Gods and Goddesses for peace. I asked them to sit with me while I continued to navigate my own fear and humanity. I focused on my breath and how simple it can really be.

All I could think about was how blessed I was to be with my babies. Yes, I know they are nine and eleven but I am their mother; they will always be my babies. How quickly life really can change in twenty seconds; how rapidly we can be jolted into the reality of our own mortality.

In a moment, the prior two days flashed before my eyes. I had made a commitment to live and share this practice of yoga from a deeper place. A place that speaks to my heart so deeply and yet, I am unsure as to why, exactly.

I promised to dive deeper into the practice of healing Mother Earth and balancing the divine feminine and sacred masculine in everything I do. I was privileged to share yoga with some amazing, loving souls just hours earlier in Golden Gate Park and the day prior in Ashland, Oregon.

I asked the yogis, *"What sings to your heart? You must share and you must share now. Mother Earth needs us all to share our gifts."* Yes, exact words.

So I was stunned and, really, taken a little aback at this earthquake. I felt, honestly, like She was saying through tears and temper tantrum, "I'm so upset... and so scared! Someone listen to me! " What an affirmation of my own personal cry for a deeper meaning.

Everything about our way of being is completely out of balance. We have been running on a system that has been focused on monetary gain, egoic evolution, patriarchal standards of excessive consumption, and industrial development without a glance or a thought about consequence.

This coupled with a general, overall suppression of the female voice, is leading our Earth to destruction. It's no one's fault... it just IS. We must embrace our ancestors for their willingness to do their best and ask for their help in healing. We must start leading future generations in beginning again with new ideas, patterns and ways of doing things. We must listen to all voices and stop the madness.

We must offer up a part of ourselves in surrender... and we must be open to receiving the gifts. We must be ready to go above and beyond and into the unfamiliar because it's about doing things differently.

And I'm not just talking about industry or politics either. I'm talking about it all. Relationships... connection... really seeing and embracing everyone. Just simply allowing the energy to exhale and love. I know you know it, Mother Gaia can't take it anymore; she just can't. She's crying, weeping, and begging for us all to heal our wounds and help Her.

It's really easy to fall into the feminine energy, actually. It starts with living in love. It means letting go of fear. Seems simple, right? Still need more direction?

It means forgiving; letting go of the need to be right; embracing a stranger; noticing and being orgasmic about nature. It means saying, "I GET to instead of I HAVE to."

It means offering what you may not even have yet but you know it's coming. It means standing in a power bigger than yourself because none of this is about you, anyway.

It means looking at what you are doing with your life and choosing that which fulfills your soul... period. It means no more "sleeping" your life away. It means noticing love, noticing fear... and embracing it all.

We cannot know when it is our time. Earthquakes are just one way for Mother Gaia to remind us of our fragility, our mortality and our peace.

I am being called to share love on this planet and guide others to find that within themselves so they can share their love with the world. Specifically, I am focused on healing the mother-daughter lineage of pain, suffering and guilt. This is my work and it's not easy as it digs deep into my soul.

But that is the work.

It doesn't have to be huge... it can be super simple. Just look up and offer it up—a smile, a glance, your heart, your time, your hand, the truth. Trust me on this one... the time is now. I love you all so much. Please, NOTICE where you put your thoughts; NOTICE your speech; LIVE in love and grace. Please. Do something and maybe no one will even notice. But that's not the point. Make a ripple of love.

Transmutation

I've been thinking a lot about this week's theme... transmutation. It's divinely perfect, as always. And in meditation all week, I've reviewed these last few years.

You see transmutation is *a change in form, appearance, structure or nature of something.* It can be *an alchemical shift of who you are and how you show up in the world energetically, emotionally, mentally and spiritually.* And in that alchemical shift that begins on the inside, we eventually take on a different form on the outside.

So, like I was saying, I have been reviewing the last few years and I'm blown away at how much I've changed. When I look at photos of myself from just three years ago, I can't get over how much I don't see my current self at all.

Not even in the least bit. It's odd really—to see a photo of yourself and feel like you are looking at a stranger.

It has taken some time, some courage, and some grieving and struggling. More than anything else though, it has taken love to be here now.

Self-love, unconditional love, tough love... you name it, it all dissolves into love.

And, in this moment where I stand right now, I remember so vividly—as if it were yesterday—when that alchemical shift started inside my heart.

> *It was a cry so subtle, but came up consistently in* Eka Pada Rajakapo-tasana *that I struggled and cried every time I would enter it. It was a cry that got louder in* Ustrasana. *My yoga practice was the beginning of my alchemical shift that has brought me here; and it's what keeps me shifting every single day.*

We are not stagnate beings; in fact, we are 75 percent water. We are supposed to shift and change... A LOT! That can be really scary for a lot of people. I mean, what would we do if things were different when we woke up in the morning? EEEK!

What's really cool, when I look back just two years, and then five years, is that the change in my personal life hasn't shifted immediately. I remember thinking it would. I remember assuming that if I simply stated that I was ready for a change, it would happen exactly when I wanted and how I wanted it to work out.

Yeah, not so much.

It happened just like the books say... in a time-lapse, slow-motion crazy sort of way that is different every time you look back at the unfolding of it all. Because that's how it works. It isn't up to you. The only thing that is up to you is the willingness to shift and expand.

For real.

It's a willingness to see magic, believe in your path, and trust in the unknown. It's a vulnerability to love and a readiness to create a grandiose life outside of your own imagination.

I remember, when I was twenty-one years old, I said I wanted to write a book about how you live your life in chapters. And how they are always leading you to the next one and the next one and the next one. I haven't written that book just yet, but I sure am living it. The odd thing is... every chapter ends in love and begins with wonder.

The Womb of Mother Earth

It started out as a chance meeting of two priestesses in Tulum. I walked into a New Moon Circle at a random place on the ocean. And my dear sister Ebyan from San Francisco was leading it. We both cried, hugged and were shaking at this chance meeting, knowing in our bellies that this was no mistake.

Ebyan asked me to smudge everyone before they walked into the temple, and this to me, was not only an honor, but also a sign. You see, I have been asking what is next for me? What is my highest calling? And this... this magical encounter pointed at me with such clarity that I could only step into it gracefully.

It was in moments like these chance meetings, symbolic circumstances, miraculous encounters and countless visits by spirit animals that I knew I had to take heed to what was happening in this magical place of Tulum.

The ritual ceremony was amazing and healing, to be sure. In the past, I may have cried, felt less than whole or felt like I needed something from this circle. This time, that was not the case. I was so in my body, in my breath and so very present to it all. I felt like a priestess, holding space for these souls.

At the end of the ceremony, when the participants left, we all sat around the altar, like wise-women and old friends, loving on each other. Grateful we had crossed paths and to share such a sacred circle.

I spent most days staring at the ocean, drinking from a coconut, and turning over so I wouldn't get burned. Not once did I feel guilty or like I should be doing something else. That was the old way of being. I felt very comfortable doing nothing but yoga, eating healthy food and napping.

My last full day there, my dear friend Ebyan asks me to go to a Cenote with her. I have no idea what it is and I agree. She has no idea where she is going, but we will figure it out. We are goddesses after all! A new sister named Summer joins us and as we are leaving she says, "Hang on, let's grab Lo"—another dear priestess sister living here in Tulum.

When she steps into the car with us, I can't help but laugh because really, it's like I'm in a movie. A really, really great movie that I could never have choreographed myself. We drive for what seems like forever because well, we're looking for a white, hand-painted sign on the left side of the road. We drive past miles and miles and miles of lush, green trees and all we're looking for is a white, hand-painted sign. That's all we are looking for.

After many chants and songs later, the sign shows up. We are so excited but when we pull up, there is a barbed wire fence telling us it's closed. This is after about an hour in the car that was supposed to be thirty minutes. That's the other thing about Tulum. I swear time stands still. It's like you're in a time warp. All the time. And not one person has any conception of time either. They say, five minutes and it's twenty. They tell you a fifteen-minute walk and it's two.

We stand there in awe of this sign, potentially halting our adventure. But not one of us hesitates. We're going anyway.

I get out of the car and realize that somewhere along the line I lost a flip-flop: either at the gas station or the fruit stand, I'm not sure which, but it's certainly gone. So the Universe decides that if I am to go at all, I will be walking barefoot. The priestesses decide to walk barefoot with me. It's as if we are on a pilgrimage. Each of us from different places on the planet, each with a different story and each of us at different points on our journey. All brought together for some magical reason to be revealed at some point. Some of us will meet later; for some of us, this will be our only experience together.

We cut a banana leaf from the nearby tree for our offerings—an avocado and a bit of fruit—and off we go. Each of us takes turns holding the barbed wire up for someone else, so we can get through this barrier, and we begin walking. With no shoes. On a gravel road.

It starts hurting, so we tell stories. We talk about all the ancestors before us who must have done something just like this but under much harsher conditions. We notice butterflies, we take photos, and we start singing. We each take a turn chanting from our own lineage, teaching each other songs to connect but mainly to stop thinking about how bad our feet hurt. We find a butterfly barely alive and take it as an offering with us to the Cenote. We have no idea how far it is; we just keep walking.

We must have been quite a sight.

As we are chanting *Hanuman Bolo*, we hear a car coming up. My first thought is one of fear. Are we going to get into trouble? Are they going to arrest us? This lovely, smiling face pulls over to us and in a blend of Mayan and Spanish, he begins to tell us that he and his brother are working on the Cenote and that is why it's closed. Lo speaks to him in Spanish and tells him that we are on a pilgrimage; she tells him about our path, and why we're there. He offers us a ride as we are still fairly far away especially on bare feet.

Now his brother pulls up on his motorcycle and smiles at us. So we get in, Summer gets on the back of the cycle, and off we go to the Cenote.

I haven't felt that alive, that connected to Source, to the Now, than I was in those moments. It reminded me of some twenty years ago when I went backpacking in the Southern Hemisphere!

He parks at a hand-painted sign that says, ENTRA CENTOE. We walk along this path that is soft to the feet, followed by Juilo and his brother and a three-legged dog, barking at us, showing us the way as if to say, "I'm so glad you are here!"

We come upon the Cenote and I peer over the edge. My eyes are in awe, my heart in a state of knowing that this is It. We arrive at the steps to get down and my jaw drops. I want to get down on my knees and bow to this magnificent, phenomenal, miracle... this Cenote, this hole in the ground that is unexplainable.

I had never seen anything like this in my life. It was as if Mother Gaia was reminding me just how precious She is. As if she was revealing herself, naked and raw, as if to say, please, please remember how special I am and please, please educate the people and the next generation so we all may experience healing. See into my womb, into my being, into the depths of me and remember who I am. Examine and know that seeing me is a blessing and privilege. Feel into me and connect with my vibration. Please take this with you... know that you are whole and share this story with others. Bring them here so they may remember.

Even now as I write these words I am crying. With gratitude, with joy, with grace and with honor.

It felt as if I was in the womb of the Great Mother Herself. As if I was swimming inside the water of her womb and bathing myself in the most cleansing waters accessible. I looked up from the descent into her vastness and was in even more awe. Was this really happening? The roots from these tress, still being fed by her, the rocks taking on different patterns now that they were exposed to the elements outside the womb. Her imperfect, perfections glistening in the sun.

We swam, we sang, we meditated, we offered her our gifts and we laughed so loud. We saved a bird who had fallen out of her nest and left her with one hundred Oms to bring her back to life. These brothers, who we lovingly named Tweedle-Dee and Tweedle-Dum, were 100 percent Mayan we found out after sharing food with them. They showed us the crystals in the walls of this amazing place and explained to us where the offering table was and that we had actually sat just above it to sing. They told us stories, took selfies with us and swam and tried to speak our language. Then they called the owner of the Cenote to tell him about us.

The brothers told the owner, Pedro, that they had never seen anything like this, and that he had to come right away. Four goddesses had shown up to bless this space. Pedro showed up to thank us, to bless us and sing with us. I still to this day, am in awe of the magic from that afternoon. The gathering, the knowing, the blessing and the grace. This was such an example of the Sacred Masculine supporting the Divine Feminine in her work to connect with Mother Gaia. We had to go through a few initiations to get there but when we did, we were blessed beyond words.

We had all hoped for a Cenote experience that was free from tourists. We didn't expect a private viewing, a personal escort, or the magic that we encountered.

And as I continue to vacillate between gypsy and grounded momma, my path became very clear in that afternoon. I am a teacher of teachers, a guide for young girls, and a priestess that holds space for women. And I do this by consciously collaborating with other amazing women around the globe.

We align with each other and remind each other of our magical powers, not by competing or trying to do it all ourselves. But instead, by uplifting each other and accompanying the beauty in each other. By supporting each other in growth and expansion. We perceive Mother Earth as sacred and witness the truth of what is happening on this planet and we offer our services to help heal. And we do this together, now.

That day, in the Womb of the Mother, I recognized my wholeness. I left behind a part of me, knowing that She would transmute the old through rebirth and regeneration. Words cannot begin to describe the feeling, the connection or the emotion that imprinted my heart, mind, and soul that day. In storytelling, I hope to convey the deep meaning of being in the now, loving what is, and paying attention to every single connection we are offered in one day.

It's amazing what can happen when you look up from your phone, get off the ride, stop thinking about what everyone else is doing and press the pause button.

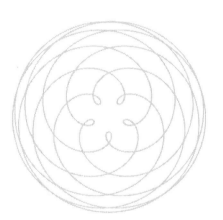

CHAPTER 4

Love and Compassion
Anahata Chakra

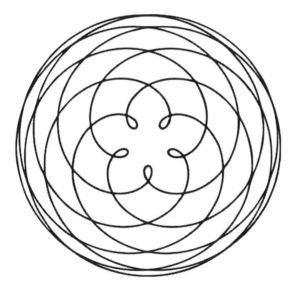

Availability

I have to be 100 percent honest and tell you that it is almost midnight and I am putting this blog together after a very full day of play dates, shopping, swimming, errands and work—yes all in a day's "work." Which makes me laugh because I get to call this all work... How blessed I am.

As I write this, know that I am not being vulnerable... no, I am being available. Available and open to the connection and resonance that will come from this blog. Vulnerable, according to my dear friend Cameron Shayne, is "living on the edge of injury," and last time I checked, I am nowhere near the edge of injury. In fact, I feel quite invincible and connected and loved and in the flow.

Availability. What are you available and ready to experience right now? I love sharing things like this; not because I am vulnerable but because I understand the power of my thoughts and my words. And I know, beyond all knowing that when I state them, courageously, from a place of insight and intuition, I am ushering in just THAT... and quickly.

This can create havoc in one's life if they are unsure of what they want, what they are capable of, or what they truly deserve, so I caution you to use your words wisely with a deep awareness on the specifics. Because it, whatever *it* is, will come charging to you... and I mean it.

So I ask you... not what you are going to state here with vulnerability, but what are you available and ready to receive?

Here's mine:

I am ready and available to receive daily downloads and insight that guide me courageously on my path.

I am ready and available to receive the support necessary to make Girls Elevate a national brand and REVOLUTION on this planet!

I am ready and available to receive the most amazing partner who has his own passion, purpose and love for life! We swoon and inspire and love on each other every, single day!

I am ready and available to receive deep presence and awareness around the profound teachings of being a mother. I know that this is the most important job I have on this planet and I am open to guidance, protection and love every bit of the way.

I am ready and available to BE a vessel for change, expansion and growth in all areas of my life.

Yes... that's all there is to say now. Yes.

State it like you mean it.

From somewhere near San Francisco:

Breathing really deep as I acknowledge the beauty, grace and amazingness in my life. So much coming into focus with such clarity and inspiration.

My prayer for this moment: Good God, continue to grace me with clarity of mind, purity of heart and consciousness of actions while I navigate the blessings bestowed upon me moment after moment after moment.

Continue to give me the clarity needed to discern what fulfills my highest purpose and passion and help me to choose what serves my calling.

Keep myself and my children wrapped in your blessings while we navigate this life creating trust in our "pod," growth and elevation in our community, and a REVOLUTION on this globe!

Compassion Is an Inside Job

"Compassion is not a relationship between the healer and the wounded. It's a relationship between equals. Only when we know our own darkness well can we be present with the darkness of others. Compassion becomes real when we recognize our shared humanity."

Pema Chödrön, *The Places That Scare You:*
A Guide to Fearlessness in Difficult Times

I love this quote. So much so that I have been reading it in class all week long, in the morning when I wake up, and before I go to bed. The world needs more compassion. I know how prophetic that sounds, but it's true. And, despite what you might think, compassion has to be an inside job.

Compassion is not "needing to understand" anything about or even why anyone does anything that they do. We can judge all we want. We can make assumptions. We can project our own ideas about why... but guess what? We know nothing. We have not walked a minute in anyone else's shoes **so we know nothing**. Best to just hold space.

The other thing is... you are perfect. Which means, so is everyone else. You are not here to fix anyone. You are only here to love them. In all their imperfections, you are here to love them unconditionally. And oh, by the way, no one needs to fix you either, so stop looking for that outside help. Remember, compassion is an inside job.

I love that she says, *"Only when we know our own darkness well can we be present with the darkness of others."* This is so important. Know thyself. Know what you love, what you live for, what you'd die for, and what triggers the shit out of you. Because your trigger is your greatest gift. It's the key to compassion. If it's still triggering you, it's something to look at with the eyes of compassion. FYI, if it's triggering you, it's not outside of you. It's inside.

You know, to be completely transparent, I spent this whole week not sitting in loving compassion for the amazing life I get to participate in. No, I spent it being triggered for a moment, and yes only a moment by my mother, my ex-husband, and my former lover. I spent it looking into the mirror asking the question,

"Where am I exhibiting this behavior? How can I shift my reality? What is real for me? How can I still love this person? And what is beautiful about this relationship that has evolved me?"

Here is what I found:

You can experience deep love and compassion while still being able to carry on a relationship, even if it looks different than what you want.

It is possible to see the bigger picture and make decisions from that place as opposed to reacting in a moment.

And sometimes, you just have to let go in deep love for yourself because their energy field just didn't resonate with you any longer.

Personally, self-compassion and self-love won and propelled me into creating boundaries for myself that had to be established in response to this shift in my own reality. **They** didn't need to change; my response had to change is all.

One of my favorite teachers says, *"There is nothing you can do to make me love you any more than I already do. And there is nothing you can do that can make me love you less. I simply love you."* You know where you start reciting that? Yup, in the mirror... today. Start there.

Connection

I've been sitting with this idea all week long and it's been a little challenging. You see, the idea of connection came to me when I sat at San Dominican University last weekend, on a beautiful Saturday afternoon, to pay tribute to a special young man I had only just begun to know.

It boggled my mind that he felt disconnected enough to take his own life. It didn't add up as I looked around the chapel of some 300 young people, all gathered in support of each other, crying and offering prayers to the family. It didn't make sense to me at all. And it made me so very, very sad... for a really long time... on a really deep level.

It wasn't like I knew him for a long time... I barely knew him at all, actually. But what I did know, I adored. His vibrancy and sweet hugs every single time we exchanged space was so special. I am lucky enough to meet so many people in my day-to-day and this one, this one I remembered. He had such a sweet disposition and would always have something kind to say.

You know... we can recite as many meditations as we want about how we are all connected. We can talk about how "going inward" is the way to connect. And how offering up a smile or hello to a stranger can make a huge difference in someone's day or maybe even their life. But it really hits home when a friend or acquaintance takes their own life.

There's a disconnect and it haunts me.

So here's what I'm offering up. A deep turn of the heart toward connection.

Connect with your family—your kids, partner, siblings and parents.

Connect with a stranger, a neighbor, a friend.

Connect with nature.

Connect deeply with your lover.

Connect with your Divine Source.

We are here to connect... period. And it doesn't happen through these little electronic devices that have become appendages, either. Connection isn't through an electromagnetic field... emanating from your phone or the computer. That actually robs you of true connection.

Connection is from the heart.

It's a look in the eyes.

It's a hand on someone else's heart or shoulder.

It's listening intently while someone else talks.

It's deep and it's real and in this technological age, it's harder to come by.

But you know what... there is nothing like it. And nothing you can tell me will make me change my mind... not one thing. I don't care who you are...

life is meant to be lived, and loved and adored through the eyes of our soul and the beating of hearts.

Please... however you do it, just do it. Put the phone down and look up. Look up at yourself in the mirror, at the stranger crossing the street, at the person bagging your groceries, at your children, at your life and at infinite space... it's all up. Look up...

Devotion

Devotion is defined as "love, loyalty, or enthusiasm for a person, activity, or cause."

I define it as something that takes your breath away. That makes time stand still. That fills your heart with expansion.

It feels like an abundance, an overflowing of love and of all resources.

It is not free from challenges, or pains, or uncomfortable-ness. No, devotion holds everything.

Devotion gives you super-human powers to go beyond; to see clearly; to live in the realm of nothing that holds everything. To live in the unknown because in that unknown, everything makes sense. To live in the darkness knowing that the light will shine when it is time.

Devotion breeds unconditional love, acceptance and integrity. And, it's fueled by an inner compass that is, indeed, indescribable. Our devotion defies gravity, logic, reasoning and sometimes universal laws. It needn't make sense. We can't possibly understand the logic of the heart because it's more intricate that our brain, so how could we understand it?

Sometimes we are told what to be devoted to. You know, that can't happen because no one lives in our own personal heart of hearts. No one can hear the song of our heart except ourselves; only we know what we are devoted to. We may try to be devoted to someone else's path or idea but really, it is our own that will keep calling us back.

We may stray when things are blurry or we are in a state of fear or confusion. That's okay. Because in that straying we learn; we gather and we observe other ways of doing things or portals into something new that sparks the heart and sends it back to its path.

Sometimes we stray because we are so afraid of the transparent vulnerability that comes with devotion, that we must look away. The light of devotion illuminates everything and until we are okay with this light and what shadows it creates, we will continue to live in mediocrity.

Devotion is the only way to live fully. Being devoted to a moment. To a breath. To presence. To your partner, to your children, to evolving, to expanding, to learning, to loving unconditionally.

To loving it all, without putting anything outside of that ring of love. To holding space for it all and allowing yourself to fall into everything that has brought you to this moment.

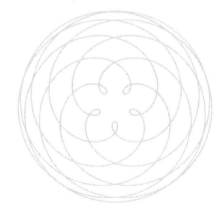

Exposure

Upon returning from Burning Man in 2015, I had a really hard time adjusting to this "default-world" that you hear Burners talk about. I wrote about this challenge just five days after returning.

What a flipping default world it is. That phrase holds so much meaning and makes me laugh out loud now. And transitioning myself from an existence where people hug, connect, love, kiss, share infinite time, help each other, share truths, and fly by their intuition into this "default reality" of schedules and work and kids and sports and "to-do's" really has this recovering Type A annoyed.

And I have an AMAZING life with EPIC changes coming up that I am so excited about! And in this moment, still, I am annoyed. Guess I am still struggling with "embracing it all."

Not to mention that I left my heart on the Playa... Literally. Left it, exposed as it's ever been. Ever. I've never loved in a moment as I did that sunrise on the Playa. Shiva-Shakti in all its glorious balance. I am so grateful to be reminded about my manifesting skills. My heart is still raw and open to what was to be, or not to be. I do not know, but I must trust. All the stars say I must trust, so I do—without worrying, planning, scheming, or unconsciously manifesting.

I want to write about exposure, the theme for the week. However, I must write about it all. Yes, all of it.

I must touch on the divine timing of all of this. The new moon in Virgo, asking for organization. And Jupiter, wanting to create a bigger container than we may be comfortable with, because it's not ALL pretty.

The solar and lunar eclipses coming up that will give us all a portal for expansion, endings, and beginnings. The way we are all manifesting at such a rapid rate that it is IMPERATIVE that we are awake to our truth. The fact that nothing is more important right now than your spiritual practice and plugging into what connects you to Source. And to the unwavering FAITH and TRUST that is necessary right now in this crazy, mystical shit storm that is realigning us with our truth and deepest desires.

Because the truth is that the Universe is asking us ALL to expand beyond what we intellectually believe we can achieve. We must all drop deeply into our intuition and be free from the constraints of what "makes sense." Maybe that means pulling the plug, for some; and maybe it means just changing the way you do things by five degrees each day.

I must remember that "Just as any creative project begins with a blank slate, your life as a creative project will unfold in its right timing with power and purpose as long as you practice unwavering Faith and Trust every step of the way."

I have a lot to say, honestly, and I think that I want to preface it all by saying that every single person on that Playa had a different experience. Burning Man is a vortex of individual experiences that are necessary for the evolution of each participant. If they are open to it.

So, while I write my own, personal, raw, vulnerable musings, please hold your tongue and your judgments, and just sit with my experience. Because if we "Burners" sit long enough, we will all see what we are meant to learn individually and how that ripples into the collective. So that's all I'm doing here.

When I first was offered the opportunity to attend Burning Man, all I could think about was how great it would be to "get it off my bucket list." To be able to teach yoga at the base of The Woman was quite an honor for this Midwest Yogini. "I just need to go once," were my words, I think.

But, you know what; Burning Man will never get crossed off my bucket list. Burning Man is now part of me, something I will never be able to give up, cross off, or forget. Burning Man is a love, a conquest, a reboot, a complete recalibration of my soul. A reminder of who I am at my deepest level. Each experience is personal, unique and potent. Now I see why so many people flock. It's what we all crave, whether we want to admit it or not.

We all want to expose ourselves from our most primal place. We all want to dance in the dust, wear little or no clothing, love each other, and do what we want, when we want. We all want to be able to honestly let go of our grip... on everything. We all want to embrace our insecurities and love them. None of us enjoys being on a timeline, a deadline or ruled by time at all. But a sweet friend said to me while I was there...

"Time is a just a grid on the Playa. It's just a place where you live."

Everyone wants to believe in magical encounters, in destined love, in a tribe, in their intuition, in their ability to be alone. Everyone wants to be transparent, authentic, and to feel intimate connection with another soul. Everyone wants to wander.

No one wants to be tethered to their damn phones; no one wants to listen to notification after notification beep on their iPad or computer. And no one wants to compete with one another. We have just been conditioned, or "defaulted" to believe that as truth.

I found Burning Man to be one of the most epic adventures of my life thus far. And I've had a lot of adventures, to be sure. This one exposed my heart, my truth, my fears, my distractions, my primal goddess in all her forms. My Shakti power at work creating, destroying and manifesting a life that is so incredible. Burning Man ignited a spark that will burn for quite awhile, amidst the to-do's of my amazing life with my two kids, this environment of San Francisco and the North Bay, the yoga school, my non-profit and the gathering of conscious people.... I am re-sparked.

I mean, really... pretty lovely.

But, here's the deal... if I had to pick one word, just one word to share for this week, it would be *exposure*. I exposed myself way beyond my comfort zone. I hate camping! Despise it! Cannot stand getting in a tent let alone with an inch of playa dust in it. I can't stand the cold, hate it. My ideal vacation is lying on the beach, coconut in my hand, getting up in between naps and lovemaking to jump in the ocean and maybe eat some food.

I exposed myself to not knowing, to harsh elements out of my control, to my fears, to my most uncomfortable places and... you know what? I noticed everything about myself and I loved it. I loved the exposure. I loved the innocence, the vulnerability, the noticing. I loved seeing all sides of me and knowing that I am not perfect, nor do I want to be.

But I do want to expose more of myself. I want that feeling on a daily basis. I want to feel primal and in alignment with all that is real. I don't want to fall into the default world. I want this truth of Burning Man to be a bigger part of the default world. Where people hug, and love, and don't give a shit what anyone else thinks. Where people see the bigger picture of life and our deepest connection.

Expose yourself just a little bit and you can be a contributor to that reality. A reality where we all love, and appreciate, and dance and sing and truly see what is real.

Who's with me?

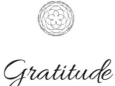

Gratitude

I write about gratitude a lot it seems. Actually, it's a great topic to revisit because in my humble opinion, it's easy to forget to be grateful. It's easy to get caught up in the drama or mundane activities in life and forget to give thanks.

And then, of course, there is the age old, "you cannot attract anything new into your life until you are grateful for what you already have."

And how about changing your verbiage from, "I have to do this, that and the other thing," to "I get to do this, that and the other thing?" That was a big one for me.

Carolyn Myss says, "Everything beyond the breath is a gift." What if we could wake up and remember that all day long? That the sheer fact that we woke up and had another day in this body was an epic gift.

I live life with no regret because I know that everything happens for a reason. I believe that this production we call our life is created to bring us home to our soul. And I believe it happens in ways we understand and ways we don't. But to separate events into categories of good or bad, or helpful or not helpful would be a disservice to the magic of it all. We must be grateful for everything.

Everything.

But I would like to explore another idea around gratitude that I'm not sure I have explored before. It's the idea about how we define gratitude. And by that, I mean specifically, how do you show gratitude? How do you receive gratitude when it comes your way? Because I think this is important.

Some people keep gratitude journals. Some people meditate in the morning giving thanks for it all before it's happened. Some people write thank-you notes. Some hug tightly and love deeply. Some display grandiose gestures of gratitude by buying gifts and out-of-this-world offerings. Others give thanks and then pay it forward.

I hesitate to tell anyone what to do... ever. But in this case, I find a combination works nicely. Whatever your way of being in gratitude, the most important thing to remember is to actually feel gratitude.

More precisely, embody the feeling of gratitude, because our emotions drive everything.

Do you know what gratitude feels like? If you don't, start feeling it now.

I feel it in my heart. My heart expands and then I notice my breath. My breath feels like particles I could see in front of me if I had on special glasses. My limbs tingle. My connection to Source comes alive. I feel like time has stopped and I'm in a vortex of swirling love. And I feel it when I am offering up gratitude and when I am receiving it... there is no difference.

You see, in my opinion, the feeling of gratitude gives us that connection to the higher realms of consciousness. We know we are connected and it's a like a rush through our bodies that is really unexplainable.

If we dig a bit deeper into gratitude and we really feel it, we can begin to recognize the true abundance in our production, in our life. And we not only receive that gift/gesture in gratitude, but we can't wait to give it away. We can't wait to be in the flow of giving and receiving all at once.

We are in the flow of life and everything begins to create itself as if by magic. Not only that, but we truly recognize that there is no separation or difference in anything. That everything that is happening is perfectly and divinely orchestrated. And that all we have to do is set intentions that mean something, give them just enough attention, and then sit back in gratitude for everything we have and are experiencing already.

That's it. Know how you show gratitude. Understand how you receive gratitude. And then get in the flow.

The Heart Knows

I was suffocating
Couldn't sleep
Totally triggered
Couldn't take it anymore
The noise, the harsh weather, the no sleep

I yearned for home

I got on my bike and rode out to the end of the world
Where I could get some perspective
I rode to where there was some space
I turned and saw how small things really were
My shadow taller than life and I could breathe

And then I saw you

And my heart opened, totally exposed
You were like a mirage in the desert
Your kindness was that of an angel
It was so simple
And I knew things were all right

The next morning I rode around in awe
The art, the life, the love
I stopped and wept many times

I offered love and forgiveness
I prayed for a new reality
I dropped it all, the pain, the grief, the disappointment

Every morning was different
An abundance of reverence and awe
Every last bit of grief, sadness, disappointment, gone
But the temple beckoned me for one more trip inside

And there you were

In a sea of people, there you were
So sweet
So sexy
So comfortable
So familiar

How could it be anyone else?

I was an adorned princess
A queen taken home
Conversation was easy and light
I laughed more than I had in years
The lines on my forehead relaxed

I was confident and content
I needn't be anything, I was everything
My soul was singing
We had found each other amidst an ocean
We knew it so we played with it

So innocent and light

I relaxed and watched magic unfold
Story after story
Truth after truth
Encounter after encounter

That evening, looking for you, I trusted and waited
I gazed into the dark
Into the flickering neon lights
Into the blazing fire
Into the writhing, dancing bodies
Listened intently for a sign
Stopped and called you in with my thoughts

Still nothing

I surrendered to the not knowing
To the not seeing
To the not embracing
And I trusted

And at the last minute there you were

In the dark
Moving swiftly
My heart leapt over the bikes and embraced you
Beyond time, space and reality

We found each other again

The embrace was breathless and so necessary
Even now my heart expands exponentially
To find that love, that grace, is a gift
Not everyone cracks their heart open
Not everyone feels the lightness of soul love
Not everyone understands connection over dimensions
Throughout stories, space, reality and time

The comfort, familiarity, the love
All real
All right
All divine—yes, divine
Two souls reunited

My heart sang and joy filled my body
We rode to camp
To the fire, to the warmth
On cue, magic showed up in the desert
And offered us shelter and comfort
To sit, to gaze, to know
To feel, to laugh, to hold
To share space and be

Your touch ignited such passion
It was like no other before
My body released without a touch
Just you next to me was enough

Despite the cold I was warm
Your embrace so safe and so familiar

My coat our only shelter

Time stood still
We traveled dimensions
Our heart and soul merged
As Venus stationed direct our bodies laid together still

You confirmed that
My work had been complete
That my karma fulfilled
Shiva manifest in this lifetime
My light reignited not just sexually
But fully
Unconditionally
The final locks on my heart open
Exposed, raw and real

When we parted
Our gaze impenetrable
We knew it wasn't over
This wasn't the end
The letting go was necessary
In grace, in gratitude, in prostration
I bowed to the gift of such a short meeting
That seemed to defy time, space and distance

The heart full
The body satisfied
The soul knowing

We meet still at the edge of reality
We sing, dance, gaze at the stars
We have sex and love make
We hold each other and share stories
We laugh and laugh and laugh
Infinite embrace

We know that we found home.

Love

I love love... I mean I really love LOVE! I've been accused of overusing the word in some of my circles. Regardless of that, I continue to use it because it rolls off my tongue and feels good when I say it.

"Love." "I love you." "I love my life."

Love has been around forever... Love has been a part of you since the second you were conceived. The minute you were created by the heavens, you became love. Love is infinite and so is the energy from the heart. The heart was formed first when we decided to incarnate. Think about that for a hot minute. When doctors look for a baby nestled in the womb, the first thing they search for is a heartbeat. Even that thought takes my breath away and brings a tear to my eye. I still remember the first time I heard the heartbeat of my two children. It is a miracle, honestly.

The heart.

It is the epicenter of everything. It holds everything. From the second we are alive in our mother's womb, we begin feeling. We felt our mother's heartbeat, her indecisions, fears, joys and desires. Immediately, our heart started writing stories that we carry, for at the very least, this lifetime.

When we were born, we yearned for our mother's breath, her touch and reassurance. That relationship sets the tone on how we define love. Our heart seeks love... our bodies crave touch. It's a fact. This feeling of love and intimate touch evolves as we get older and we seek out partnerships to fulfill that need, but the fact is, we are meant to feel and love another.

But I'd like to add something that I can't prove, I just know it—it's in the fabric of my being and yours too. If love is infinite, wouldn't it be safe to say that even before we incarnated, we were love? That we already came in knowing that we were divine love? That, before we were even born, we were love. I don't know for sure, but when I sit and feel into that, it feels right.

I mean, when you feel something that frustrates you, hurts you, or creates contraction in the body, it is not love. And you know it. Whether or not you pursue it is based on your patterns. As you move along this path of life you are continually defining and redefining love and what it really means to you based on how you feel.

The heart is a beacon, it knows truth and it vibrates YOUR truth. And throughout your life, your heart has been nurtured, filled up, stepped on, mended, broken, ignited, full and then empty again and again. It is this amazing vessel of infinite capacity.

Your heart laughs, cries, embraces and screams. Think about it... it does so much. And, by the way, it beats and keeps you alive without you having to do a thing.

Another tidbit: The depth of hurt your heart has held acts as a springboard to catapult your heart into an immeasurable feeling of love and gratitude. So, the deeper your hurt, the more capacity you have to rebound into love that skyrockets.

Yes, we are molded by our mother's patterns and thoughts on love. Yes, we draw in ideas and fantasies about love with every relationship that we witness from the time we are born. Yes, we fall "into" love and stumble around blindly when the feeling of love envelopes our heart. Yes, we crumble when love ends in abandonment, or neglect or is not reciprocated. But the heart is infinite... it knows love. It knows that it can always repair itself. It just has to go inward and heal.

This is what I know to be true:

- My heart broke many times throughout my childhood.

- My heart filled up when I got married many years later.

- When I write about love or connection, it flows off my fingertips without thought.

- Love flows from me every time I step on my mat and move my body.

- My heart broke again when my marriage ended in divorce.

- When my child says, "I love you, mommy" my heart leaps and almost explodes.

- When I watch my children in a dance recital or school function, I cry—every single time.

- When I look deep into the eyes of my lover, I see love from his heart—our love connection, and it's magic.

- But most importantly... when I look into the mirror and see myself, I see love.

Beyond the fear, guilt, hurt, shame and mistakes and beyond the paths I've taken that led nowhere, past the indecisions and decisions I made that turned out different than I expected, I am love. We all are.

At the foundation of it all, you are love. Alone. You aren't love WITH someone... you're just expanded love when that union happens. Alone... just you... you are love: infinite love to be exact.

I am done skimming the surface of life, moving and breathing from a place that only excites my body and my mind. Let's excite the heart! Rewrite patterns that put fear before love! Let's put love first! Let's give the heart a chance to feel into the depths of the pain so it can come up for air fully healed and ready to lead you to more love!

Revisit whatever it is fully and then come up for air.

We are waiting with open arms.

Love for My Father

I have waited all week to write this blog. It's super painful and I haven't really been up for it, to be honest. I have pushed this aside and anguished over my feelings around this for years... literally years.

I had every intention of writing it on Father's Day, in honor of my father. However, I just couldn't do it. It's time now, though, because... as I look at my life... my relationships with men, in particular, I realize that in order for me to move completely forward, this has to be out in the open.

Not only that, as I watch my young daughters grow into young women, I find that it is more important than ever for them to understand how powerful love between father and daughter really is.

I never had that relationship with my dad. And as a woman in this world, I don't know if you really ever get over not having a relationship with your father, especially when you lived under the same roof for a good sixteen years of your life.

My dad was a man in pain. He was angry all the time. He was never really around. He treated my mom less than she deserved, and abused my sister and I verbally, emotionally and physically. I watched all this. As a child of God, I watched it all and never understood any of it.

I wanted his love so badly, as any daughter does, but it just wasn't there. At least not in a way I could understand. Through the yelling, then him slamming doors and then finally leaving, I was just plain-ass scared of him. I always felt abandoned and sad. My sister used to hide in her closet.

As soon as I was old enough, I got the hell out of there. It all made no sense to me. Not his actions, not how my mother put up with it all, none of it. It put a real damper on the good things I'm sure he did because the grooves that the pain, fear and terror made in the brain, ran much deeper than bliss and love.

None of this seemingly meant a thing until I got married and had two kids of my own. I witnessed myself in pattern mode for several years and I thank God for my yoga practice. I undid lots of patterns, one at a time, like you unravel a ball of yarn: with consciousness, intention and methodology.

I learned grace, compassion, forgiveness, love, strength, intuition, appropriate use of power and the significance of harnessing your energy and moving through your feelings without numbing to it all. I was able to witness, cry through it, move through it and create new patterns. And that took time, dedication, commitment, truth and lots of hours on my mat.

I don't think my parents had this awareness. No, it was quite different for their generation. I'm from the Midwest, Italian descent, Catholic born and raised. My parents, uncles and aunts, grandparents and neighbors all drank wine with lunch and Sambuca in the evening with cigars. Old men sat on the porch; women worked in the kitchen. Yup, that's how it was. We heard our dad whistle at the end of the day and we knew it was time to come home.

And children were seen but definitely not heard.

There was a beauty to my childhood: like riding my bike everywhere; gardening with my grandmother; going to the lake in the summer; swimming at my neighbors' house all the time. A big part of it never felt quite right, but I went along with it because, really, what choice did I have? Then when I was old enough, I numbed myself for a really, really, long time. I think I was around forty when I woke up... like, really woke up, and saw what was happening.

It was hard to make a change; pulling the plug felt like chopping off my right arm. My heart hurt all the time and I thought for sure, just this once, I would have the support of my mother or my father. But, even then, I didn't. I fell into the abyss of my new life not knowing where the net was. But it appeared, over and over again without fail.

What never resonated through all of this, though, was the absence of unconditional love. I mean, true love... no matter what. And never, not once, was there an "I'm sorry" to put the salve on my child–like heart.

Now before you think, oh poor girl... let me say something. I have learned a lot. I believe life is exactly perfect. So I am not bitter. I'm like that little tomboy, falling out of trees and banging herself up, but getting right back up to do it again. I'm that girl who is friends with everyone because I AM unconditional love, I AM grace, I AM forgiveness, I AM non-judgment. Could I be that without all that experience? Perhaps not. So I am grateful.

I have to be brutally honest, though, and say this deal with my father has been my deepest wound to date that I have not been able to fully admit forgiveness with.

There are times when I want to scream and say, "What the FUCK? I was a kickass little girl! Why did you do all those things?" And believe me, I have used every tool in my toolbox; I have prayed, breathed, mantra-ed, reached out in grace, even used my kids as an excuse... name it. There was still this... this thorn... under my fingernail with this one. And it showed up several times in relationships with men.

Finally, I caught on fully, and I have a few catalysts to thank. One is my lovely daughters: I watch them love on their father and it makes me so happy. He may not be my cup of tea, but the space our divorce made allows us all to love each other as we want... no expectations, and everyone gets to be who they are.

Another reason is because I witness time—the illusion of time that turns our hair gray, makes wisdom lines on our faces and memory lapses in our conversations—and I know my father is growing old. I know he will die soon. It breaks my heart that we don't talk, but I can't do much more than I have.

And the other thing, and most likely the most important reason, is because I have longed my entire life for true love. I AM one of those people that believe in true love. I am a romantic, truth be told. It won't come if I create a barrier to unspoken unconditional love and forgiveness for the man who brought me here!

How do I tie all this together? Why do I put this out there? No, I am not afraid of what people might think. Because here is the lesson that I think is so important for everyone to understand:

> You mustn't ever give up on anyone, no matter what. You mustn't hold onto your own pain, your own anguish... it will only follow you around. AND when you give up on someone else, you are giving up on yourself. Period. Don't do that.

Conversely though, understand the power of your energy and bring forth your heart without dropping it on the floor to be stomped on, again. That does nothing but drain you. Instead know where to draw a line of what you put "out there" and then just be open to receive what comes back.

Our theme this week has been forgiveness—deep forgiveness. And although I have done work like this on many a weekend retreat, in many a yoga class and in many tearful moments at my altar, I have never put it out there for anyone else to know, to read, until now.

Between this past full moon and today's Solstice, I am ready to let my pain go... for good. I am ready to dance, to fall into love, and to experience real forgiveness for my father. I am ready to let it all go with an open door in the event he comes to me, in his own way. I will always have my arms open, my heart unguarded, my mind free from questions, from the why. This takes daily work and I know that... it's a re-aligning and redesigning of my patterns. Isn't this why some of us come here?

I am ready to love and to move forward, not looking back, ever. Not missing or wishing for what could have been. For years, I thought something was wrong with me. Nothing was wrong with anything... I came here to learn forgiveness, and that I have done.

I am ready to move forward with a strength and grace that is palpable. Swift and conscious like a deer. Nurturing and loving like a momma. Sensual and intimate like a goddess.

To all of my teachers who brought me to this power, to this strength, to this clarity and vision and who helped me see my wings, who have supported me, have loved me and who continue to stand by me... I am grateful. This one was hard. Many blessings.

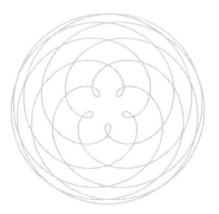

Ocean Cleanse

I went to the ocean to wash it all away. The rage, the fear, the grief, the guilt and the shame. It has been a process, to be sure, but this time was different and I knew it. I felt spirit ushering me to my highest order and deepest purpose, and I knew this trip to the beach was important. I knew that it was time to stop licking my old wounds so I could be totally present to my amazing life beyond the hurt I had swept under the rug for so very long.

I felt the water on my feet and I just knew the ocean, Mother Gaia herself was transmuting it all and cleansing this body of mine. I went there praying for healing. I went with my children because amidst all of our chaos and busyness, their innocence, presence, truth and love for life soothes my soul like nothing else.

I let wave after wave sweep over my feet, taking my past to the center of Gaia where it could be transmuted into love. I watched my daughters play and felt peace, joy, abundance and reverence for it all. I have never felt more empowered in all my life. I felt a whoosh of fresh air as my soul spoke so loudly, "This is all divine and absolutely perfect." I felt the energy in my arms release the weights I had been carrying of my past, my ancestors, and my previous lives.

How did I know I was healed?

Time stood still while I watched the super moon come up and the sun go down.

I promised myself I would get to the root of my healing and I did. That doesn't mean I'm done or I have nothing else to do in life. No, it just means that I see things now with much more clarity. It means that I witness reflection after reflection after reflection and can face them with love and honor, diffusing the projection and continuation into the next life.

I felt the hand of God at my back and the whisper of angels in my ear, "It's time to trust and listen." There is no longer room or space for anything other than truth. I experienced *santosha* like never before, to just sit and not feel like I was missing out on one single thing. This is a new one for me.

On this super moon and sunset, I set abundance and clarity into motion as I let go of my past, stay rooted and grateful for the present while I trust in what is coming in the future.

I forgive it all, especially my own ignorance in decision-making and disempowering choices.

What does this mean?

It means that I no longer need to be seen or understood. It means that I feel the hair stand up on my arms when I talk about the masculine and feminine energy rising and how we all play a part in it. It means that I have no time for small talk or games and I am not afraid to say so or set my boundaries up, either. It means that I trust that everything is happening for me in every moment. It means that, finally, I know that I am enough and that the Universe continues to provide.

I know that it is time for us all to drop our addictions, let go of our repetitive wounded stories and move forward with love, trust and grace so that we may experience freedom and justice from of the heart for generations to come.

Open the Heart

So you opened the heart, did you? You put yourself out there. You went out on that limb. And now, your heart is filled up so much that you can't help but share, enlighten, love, express and BE that love! The Universe seems to be moving along with the rhythm of your heart; you can FEEL that expansiveness and authentic connection with all that Is. Everything you think, feel and communicate is infused with love and pure gratitude.

The only thing is that it seems like everything is rushing to you at once. In fact, all of a sudden you seem like this powerful beacon, which you are, and every thought you have is manifest.

This can be really overwhelming because you would like to "have it all." But, keep in mind that having it all means managing it all, too. So when life is rushing to you, and you can feel that it's time to make some decisions, what do you do?

I mean, if you can have it all, which you can, how do you know what to choose? How do you know what's "right"? How do you know what the consequences of your decisions are going to be? How do you know what decision will make you most fulfilled?

The answer is you don't. You don't know. You can't know. You may try to line things up just so, so that things work out according to your plan but I can tell you right now, it's not your plan, it's God's.

So then how do you decide? How do you find that balance between goal-setting to get what you want out of life and allowing the Universe to guide you? This is a tough one, isn't it? Because although we think we have control over our destiny, there IS Higher Power that guides us.

Finding that balance between what WE think is best and what God thinks is best can only be realized through stillness. You find stillness. Providing that you have infused love, gratitude and compassion into your thoughts and actions, the only thing left is to be still and listen.

Clarity is NOT found in distracting yourself with mindless activities. It's not found in busying yourself with too much work, drink or other addiction. It's not found in incessantly talking about or "weighing your options." It is found in stillness... plain and simple.

That space where everything is quiet and potentially dark. Your eyes don't focus in on what step to take next, your heart does. Your heart and breath guide you authentically into stillness.

As a society we don't take that time often enough. With all the information available at our fingertips these days, finding stillness and quiet takes effort. It takes dedication and commitment. But those who take it understand the power in that stillness and come back to it repeatedly for that guidance that they know speaks from their heart.

Go ahead and set your goals. Get your eyes focused on what you believe is the right path, decision or choice for you. Do that! You are human! Then, close your eyes and listen to your heart. Allow for that graceful space of nothingness to come in and truly guide you. Ask, "What is for my highest good?" "How can I serve and use my God-given gift?" And say over and over again, "I trust, believe, I am."

You will know you are on the right path when you feel gently ushered along your path. You will know you are humming along life when you experience serendipitous moments regularly. You will know you are living through clarity when there is no struggle.

A mantra that came to me one morning in stillness was this:

> *"My life is a divine manifestation of following my heart deeper and more open in everything I do from business, relationships, yoga, parenting... All are One. Hari Om, Hari Om, Hari Om."*

Take some time... even if it's five minutes... be still... Listen... inhale, exhale, say thank you. That's it.

Relationship

This word, oh, this word. Since it came into my awareness over ten days ago, I feel like I have been run through the wringer. And it hasn't been just me either. I've been witness to emails, Facebook messages, texts and phone calls from people going through the same thing... relationship issues.

Venus in retrograde coupled with a full moon in Aquarius was a doozy of energy. And if you didn't feel it, good for you. But here's the deal, we ALL are experiencing relationship stuff; whether or not we are awake to it is a whole other story. Not only that, but the energy will come back around at some point that works for you.

Because the reality is, a full moon and Venus Dance asks us to drop it all and be the best we can be. It asks us to rejuvenate and bring to light all of our shadows because in the shadow the pearl lives and is waiting to be discovered. It encourages us to love it all and be free from what drags us down once and for all.

Beyond that, the truth is that we are all ascending to a higher vibration of love and we can't carry anything heavy or dense. We just can't! So we can either keep trying to carry it, shove it under the rug, point the finger out at someone else, or we can own it and deal with it and look it square in the eye because the time is now to love it and move on.

Because here is the deal:

We have relationships...

to others

to ourselves

to money

to social media

to food

to alcohol

to fame and fortune

to spirituality

to work

Just name it. How you relate in the world to ANYTHING, is a relationship.

Originally, I wanted to use prophetic sentences for this blog like:

Every relationship is a reflection of yourself.

Relationships are why you are here.

Relationships come and go.

I let go of relationships that no longer serve me.

The relationship I have with myself is all I need.

Yada, yada, yada... And while I believe all of that, here's a story I want to share:

One day, driving home from work, I got word from my children that their father had moved in with his girlfriend and I shouldn't be surprised when they came to visit. This brought up some very old stuff. Some deep-rooted, relationship stuff.

I found myself trying to figure out how I was going to hold space for them while they emotionally dumped on me when I got home. Thankfully, I needed to stop at Trader Joe's on the way home, which gave me space.

But what happened next surprised the heck out of this strong, warrior mom. I was bagging my groceries and I started to weep. The weeping escalated, and soon, I was crying uncontrollably at the check-out line. Poor Trader Joe's dude, he didn't see this one coming and neither did I.

The little sniffles turned into uncontrollable sobs once I exited the store, which turned into wails and rants on the car ride home. I had to pull it together before I got home, but how was I going to pull it together when I had no idea why I was falling apart?

Best advice came from a dear friend. He said, "Stop what you are doing, park your car and look in the mirror. Look and tell me what you see."

I saw a five year old who had been neglected by her dad.

A teenager who was very troubled and had nowhere to turn.

An adult who was scared to leave her marriage.

And a sweet soul who loves life and just wants everyone to get along.

And then I saw a really **vibrant, kickass queen who has surrounded herself with amazingness, power and grace.** Someone who has walked a really crazy line of truth, freedom, and love to find herself. I saw a woman who has always been in love with life even when she didn't know what the hell she was doing.

And most of all, I saw someone who has always known who she is and what she is capable of, regardless of the stories that have colored her life.

Every relationship is a story to guide us. Every story has shaped the path, the relationships we find ourselves in are here to elevate us. That's not prophetic, it's the truth.

And here's the deal...

> *As relationships come in and out of our lives, we get to dictate just how embedded we are in them and their stories. We get to say if they resonate with us. We have the right to say just how much we are defined by them. And then we can dictate just how much we are willing to put up with, vibrate alongside, or let go of.*

And then, most importantly... and I remembered this as I watched the snot drip from my nose, my eyes bulging from my head, and my heart hurting while my gut wrenched from crying in the mirror... you are light.

You are light. You are divine light, colored by relationships reminding you to BE that. There is only one relationship that can be cultivated, examined and elevated, and that is the one you have with yourself.

You can never change another or what they do in relationship.

You cannot expect anything of anyone besides what they offer up.

Breathing in moments of perceived crisis or chaos brings you to a deeper level of understanding of yourself.

That is where the truth in relationship lies.

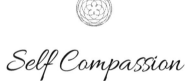

Self Compassion

You know... I looked up *compassion* because I just had to. It said:

sympathetic pity and concern for the sufferings or misfortunes of others; pity, sympathy, empathy, care, concern, mercy, tolerance

I would like to add to this. How about:

Recognizing that "you" and "I" are the same. That if we are truly living in compassion, then we subscribe to the fact that we are all One. That there is no separation and no such thing as duality. And that when we damn someone else, we are actually damning ourselves. And that when we look into the eyes of another, if we stare just long enough, we see ourselves.

Intense, I know. But very true if you sit with it long enough.

I find it very easy to feel compassion for say, a global issue that is out of my control. I can meditate on the healing of that. Easy. Even easier to love and feel compassion for those individuals outside of our sphere, a stranger on the street, a homeless person we buy a sandwich for, an arguing couple on the street.

Now try compassion for self on for size. Even better, have compassion for someone who is hurting you, disrespecting you, disempowering you, or treating you less than you deserve. How does that feel?

Ah, the frustration, resentment, hurt and feelings of separateness, how they come a calling. Harassing you to react, and react in the way you have always reacted. From a place of anger or rage or justifying your worth and stance in this situation. Because what else is there, right?

Wow. Anyone else feel that? I know I do. That's why I am a self-proclaimed work in progress.

But wait, how about if we shifted this just a bit? What if we took a different perspective on the whole thing? What if we asked, **how could this person be hurting me? There is only one of us here.** This is a holographic Universe and he is me, and she is me, and we are all One. So what the hell? Why am I bothered?

Okay, so then, when we remember that we are all one, the question becomes, **why I am creating and allowing this again? Did I not learn my lesson enough the first time? Am I not a spiritual being living this human experience in love and compassion and grace FOR ALL? FOR ALL? Not just a select few.**

Whew... Hang on. Truth: We are all one.

We do create our experiences for healing. And our core issues come up over and over again, potentially through lifetimes. That is truth. So we may experience circumstances that continually sideline us, flatten us or downright kick us to the curb.

Do not be alarmed. Even Buddha said something like, "When a mosquito bites me, I let it have its way with me. However, if it takes more than it needs or am I willing to give, I end its life."

Here's the deal:

We are all one. We do create our own experiences. We are living in a holographic Universe. And, there is such a thing as too much compassion directed down an alley that can't receive it or toward someone or something that no longer represents who we are.

Learn to direct your compassion in one direction, to Self. Because that is all there is. Self. Remember? And then notice how things shift. Be compassionate to Self. Sit in awe and wonder about who you were, who you are and who you are becoming, and bless it all. It's all a creation of your own thoughts and vibration, really. So where do you want to vibrate and ignite and create from?

What feeds you? Fuels you? Ignites you? Makes you feel good?

Do that.

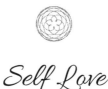

Self Love

I am not even going to tell you how much has transpired this past week of being open and available. I believe this last week was like riding a really awesome wave... at least it was for me anyway. Time opened up and, instead of filling it with "stuff to do" and "places to be," I sat.

I sat in stillness, in silence, in the quiet of my home and my heart. I did things a little differently... I got up at 5:00 a.m. and went to SoulCyle. I turned my phone off, I didn't try to make plans with people; I waited for them to reach out to me and, above all else, I took care of me. I got my hair done, my nails done, two tattoos and a massage.

I pressed a little pause button on the noise of my life and heaved a heavy exhalation. On the other side of that exhalation was space... love... grace... inspiration. To be fair, before I got to all that foo-foo... there was fear, anger, confusion, sadness, loneliness, shadows and a little darkness.

So I took a breath and sat still. Because I know that in that space of darkness and light combined, there are deep questions that try to emerge. You see, I think we ARE like onions... we are layers and layers of complexity. Anytime the space around us gets still, we are offered a revelation—a chance to peel away and get to the root—which is where the goodness lives, you know. At the root.

When we are still, open and available, and when we are truly listening, we can witness who shows up along our path and what their message is for us. We aren't waiting for them to finish so we can respond; we are truly in a state of receiving so we can transmit and integrate.

This is one powerful message that came through me this week... I've mentioned it few times and people have gasped and said, "Yes, I get that... boy I needed to hear that."

Here it is... ready?

We can manifest almost everything and anything we want or desire in this life. In fact, we are manifesting in every single second of our lives. However, we cannot manifest love... not ever. Why?

Because love must be felt from an internal place. Love comes from the inside out. It is not an emotion, or even a feeling... it is being; and it lives inside our hearts infinitely.

To understand this completely though, one must love oneself from the inside out. Once that happens fully, that self-love, then we can magnetize or attract that same love into our life. Because that love that resides within us is emanating out into the world as self-love and the only thing it can do is reflect back to us in a partner, in an act of kindness, in a shower of love from a child... You see?

That is how love manifests in our life... and, for now, I'm sticking with that, if for no other reason but to continue to love myself.

Sit in Joy

People ask me all the time, "How do you do it? How do you manifest every single thing you say you are going to do?" And I laugh because, although I've gotten really skilled at manifesting the good things, I've also been witness to patterns that create less than desirable outcomes time and time again.

So I ask you now, what are some patterns that you see happening in your life? Anything? Anything at all? Do you LIKE those patterns? Maybe they are okay but maybe not.

So let's try something really simple that, personally, I have been experiencing some amazing results with.

Ready? Sit in joy.

Yes, that's right. Sit in joy. Every single day, preferably in the morning before your day starts, close your eyes and think about one thing that makes you feel joyful. Maybe it is a past experience, maybe it's someone you love, or maybe it's something you are visualizing for your future.

How does that feel? You may feel your heartbeat, or you may get goosebumps on your arms, maybe your stomach flip-flops. Either way, FEEL joy and THEN after you roll around in THAT for a while, say thank you.

We are exposed to so much during our day, and other peoples' moods and energy can have a profound effect on our energy. It is astonishing how one person or circumstance can either really catapult you into an energetic high or knock you down into an all-time low. It's inevitable.

Unless... you manage your energy and sit in joy as often as you can.

What happens when you sit in joy?

Your world becomes your own. You manifest quicker. You radiate joy. Things don't bother you. You actually can FEEL yourself repelling (compassionately of course) those energies that do not vibrate in your field.

What happens then? You ONLY manifest that
which vibrates at your heart level.

Which is... LOVE.

Easy, right? Now go do it.

Last bit: Pass this on to someone you love AND then pass it on to someone you don't love so much. Why? Because it creates joy and that is what this world is all about.

Surrender

I've been playing around with this word *surrender* all week long and I purposely waited until Thursday night to write this because I just knew the word would completely rock my week... and it did. And let me just say here, I'm not going to skim the surface with sugar-coated, prophetic words threaded together, instead it's laced in truth.

I was a bit concerned with Kali Ma coming through so strong and ferocious; Pluto retrograde hot on her heels to stir up some darkness. Then the full moon in Scorpio begging for the death and dying of the old, so truth can prevail, all wrapped up in the shadow of Mercury stationing to go direct. That's a lot happening at one time. And, honestly, I wanted to hide; I just wanted to rest. To head to Hawaii, Mexico, Sonoma, anywhere that I could lay in the sun and let the storm pass.

But, instead, I got ready for battle.

And as I do, well, I dove right in with trident in one hand, sword in the other, just like my goddess, Durga. But this time the healing didn't come from my former pattern of masculine warrior-like actions, it came from surrendering my sword, laying down my trident and looking into the eyes of another soul so deeply that my heart hurt. It came from being so vulnerable that the words were choked up with tears the second they came out of my mouth. It was a result of finally stating what I wanted from a place that was clear, intentional and purposeful. It came from me looking at that child within myself and honoring her for all that she had gone through and finally asking for help.

I have been asking for months, for all of my old stuff to come to me so I can swallow it whole and deal with it as it comes back into my face, once and for all. I have been asking for radical forgiveness... to be able to give it and receive it. And it is here—all of it. I have to say I am in deep surrender.

Deep surrender around the fear of failing...

Deep surrender about what people think...

Deep surrender about body image...

Deep surrender about relationship...

Deep surrender around intimacy...

Deep surrender around unconditional love...

And here it all is... at my doorstep saying, "Look at me, look at me, look at me!" My head says, "No flippin' way... it's too much!" but my heart says... "BRING IT ON!"

Surrender to the heart... surrender to the heart... surrender to the heart.

The heart knows so much; it can tell stories about you from before you were born! It holds it all and it wants you to rest in it all.

Why is this hard for so many people? I don't know. But surrendering to our dark corners is the most ferocious work in this human life. It is medicine for the soul, and within our shadows lays all the light we ever need to illuminate our deepest purpose.

So when you ask me why would I do this, willingly? Resurface tears and fear and screams of anger and resentment never spoken... Why? Because I have a purpose and, if those things go unexpressed, I won't get to live that purpose in this lifetime. And as far as I know, we only get one life.

And, I'm here to live big and to love large; which means truth must prevail 100 percent of the time. Surrendering to truth isn't always easy because, quite often, it means walking through fear, guilt, shame, grief, or illusion first. But when you surrender, you relax into freedom and love. When this happens, we truly recognize that life is one magical event after another and we really aren't what we think we are... We are more.

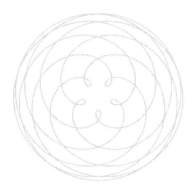

Transparency

Someone said to me the other day, "I really enjoy knowing you, Dana. Sometimes I go to class and I feel like I really don't know the teacher. I feel like I know you, and that just makes me feel good. Thank you for 'putting yourself out there' so authentically."

The funny thing about this exchange is that I have always been a pretty transparent person. I figure, I may as well lay it all out there. That way there aren't any surprises later on in a relationship—it just makes things easier, I guess. At the same time, regardless of what it looks like to you, I really despise the self-promotion this job requires. I would rather sit on my deck, in my pajamas, at my computer, writing anonymously, about life. But, too late now... I've put myself out there.

My transparency doesn't sit well with everyone, either. On a recent occasion, I was accused of "airing my dirty laundry" in my book, *Oms from the Mat*, on Facebook, *Elephant Journal*, *ORIGIN* and my own personal blog. I admit that I do enjoy telling a story. I do it, however, not from a place of boasting or needing to vent, but from a place of inspiring others.

So it got me thinking about what I really want to put out there as not only a yoga instructor but also a human being. What kind of vibe do I want to send? Who do I want to be?

My vibe came up as *approachable,* and the only answer to who I want to be was *myself.*

Here's what I came up with to share:

1. Everyone has a story.

    And you are entitled to share it in a way that works for you. For me, I bear all to inspire. Do what works for you... but do it from a place that lacks ego and exposes the heart. Period. When we tell our story, it gives others permission to do the same.

2. Go your own way.

   My decisions in life have nothing to do with yours. I hope that something I say or do inspires you in the end and that you do what your inner wisdom tells you to do. For example, my "true north" may mean dismantling my life and starting over. Yours may mean just shifting a little to the left or a little to the right in order to change your course a wee bit.

3. Don't judge your neighbor's decision.

   Why? Because it's their decision, based on their beliefs, their past and their desires... not yours. No judging please... only encouragement every step of the way.

4. Wake up to your life!

   There are miracles happening in every second and YOU are creating them. Be mindful with your words and thoughts. Set boundaries and standards that make you feel expanded and light. FEEL into your truth and then LIVE IT. Vibrate into your purpose and leave the rest behind, lovingly and fearlessly.

5. Share your story from your heart.

   Because of forums like Facebook, our ability to share our story has expanded exponentially. We grow brave "putting it all out there" because we can hide behind the computer. This is a good thing, as long as the ego is quiet. However, on some days, I feel icky about Facebook because it can feel like a "look at me" contest.

   My personal mantra with social media: *Keep sharing from your heart... not from a need to be recognized.*

6. Full frontal exposure.

   The next step to approachability and being yourself: Step on your mat and move your body in a TOTALLY unfamiliar way. Fall on your face, lose your balance and laugh a lot. I've done all those things... many times over and I am still working on handstand away from the wall. Remember, I don't want to be perfect; I want to inspire. So I continue to be real.

This is where the story ends. When I stand on my mat, I am fully exposed. People *see* me and my energy precedes my body as I walk into the room. Students have seen me on Facebook, Instagram, Twitter and they have been referred by friends. My only job is to be as clean and clear as possible energetically, so I can be approachable to students and lead the class from a place that is authentic and not riddled with ego. The last thing I want personally as a yoga instructor is to be put on a pedestal or thought to be perfect. It's too much responsibility. I just want to be me.

If you come to my class, this is what I expect:

- See yourself in me.

- Allow me to witness a nugget of myself in you.

- Be open. Laugh. Breathe... OUT LOUD!

- Do something a little out of your comfort zone just for fun.

When we do these things, we can share an intimate relationship in our yoga space without ever touching each other. All we do is breathe, move and maybe laugh a little and we are One.

Untimely Death

The death of Robin Williams brought me to tears. It wasn't because I was his biggest fan, although I do feel he was a genius living in our midst, for sure.

No, I was crying for the loss of our connection to it all—for the loss in the balance of divine order in our world. That someone so talented and lovely was tortured by so much inside and despite all his worldly things, his money, his power, his obvious love of life and people and laughter, he could not extricate himself.

This is what is heartbreaking to me.

I was crying because, being a self-proclaimed yogini, there are so many ways we can look at this and examine, and judge, and hypothesize and summarize. I mean, which came first, the addiction or the depression? Why are we as a society so focused on his depression, anyway? Why not the addiction? Why not the genetics? Was it genetic? How was his childhood? What was his home life like? Why? Why? Why?

Was this his karma? Was this his choice? If we have a choice and we create the life we want, why would he choose this? How could he not see the beauty, the glory, the blessings? What did he do in his past life that brought him here?

I mean, really, there are so many ways to examine this. And we will NEVER know the truth about his story because we did not walk his path since the day he decided to incarnate onto this planet.

But that's not our job, to know everything about this situation or even to try and understand it. Our one and only job is to hold space—space for his soul to find its way; space for his family to heal; space for the planet to exhale; space for us all to shift this energy.

I was crying, too, because the reality is that horrific things happen across this planet DAILY and we don't know about it. Why? Because the person involved was not a celebrity or "known" individual. They were a "nobody."... But they were someone to somebody, and it happens all the time.

If you must do something... because we all can, pray for the healing of all individuals on this planet and may they be well. May they embrace their light and the light of others, while embracing their dark, as well. May all beings everywhere love one another and hold space for every person to have their experience... whatever it is.

The imbalance of energy, between the sacred masculine and the divine feminine is obvious. There is a need for an up-rise of loving, compassionate energy, period. That is not to mean that we suppress, overpower, or ignore our masculine counterpart. No, in fact it is the exact opposite. We must uplift them too, for this very reason. I mean, how many men out there feel like they must "hold it together" for the sake of their family, their namesake, their livelihood. That to me is hell. Holding in your true feelings and trying to be something you're not? Hell.

The feminine energy holds space and elevates it all: the light and the dark, without judgment, or expecting or understanding.

We come to our brothers and our sisters on this planet with love and recognition that we are all in this together and we must love one another because we ARE one another.

Robin Williams' death is only one tragic example of our humanity falling from this grace and this inherent knowledge of connection. Many blessings can come of this if we all begin truly seeing this planet as a unit. As an energy that needs love and guidance and space. *That* disease, whatever dis-ease it is, has come about because of an imbalance in emotional energy within an individual, which is representative of the whole.

When energy is released and space is held for that energy to transmute, disease can dissipate. Suppressed energy is volatile and will destroy, implode or explode into something that we witness as anger, manic depression, addiction and the list goes on and on.

So here we are. What to do?

We hold space. We hold space for every single being on the planet who is suffering, and we look to ourselves for guidance on how to use our own amazing gifts to heal the planet. We examine our own dark side and see how our world can heal another. We express our creativity without defense or explanation. We step into our light and share our gifts. We uplift humanity by uplifting ourselves. We walk with grace and ease, courage and humility, power and poise, love and light.

Truly, that is all.

Breathe.

CHAPTER 5

Expression and Truth
Vissuddha Chakra

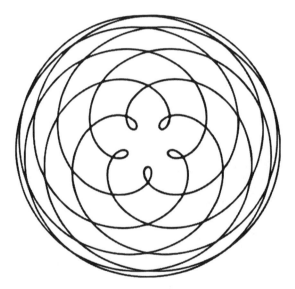

Alchemy

I'm not sure how *alchemy* landed in my lap this week as the theme, but it landed and it landed hard.

I have avoided this word for quite some time, and honestly, I'm not sure why. I think it's because I feel like a sorceress when I use the word... alchemy! And I, like anyone else, sometimes tend to be a bit timid with my powers. Especially when I start using them without really knowing how.

Alchemy... A seemingly magical process of transformation, creation or combination. The medieval forerunner of chemistry, based on the transformation of matter.

What does this have to do with yoga? What does this have to do with breath? What does this have to do with life?

Everything. So much so that I'm not quite sure where to start.

First off, when you surrender to this, this power... you realize that everything happening around you is being created by your own thoughts. And you wake up to it all. Sometimes it's almost as if my life is working in slow motion, and I think a thought and then wait for it to manifest. And now, now it's to the point that when I witness myself falling into an old pattern, some lower vibration, I literally stop what I'm doing and ask for a do-over.

Why? Because we can do that. We are transforming in every single breath and in every single moment. Why not be alive and awake to it all and then direct and consciously create your life, right?!

Secondly, the whole idea that yoga is at the forefront of human consciousness resonates deep within me and has become my lifestyle. Yoga: to yoke, to unite. To bring together breath, movement, thought, reaction. To release the stagnation in the body so you can begin to see with your inner knowing and cease to rely on the external world for guidance. That's where the magic begins... going inward.

Third and most important I think, is this: the heart. Oh my goddess, the heart. Sometimes when I drop into the energy of the heart, I cry. Not because of pain but because I can feel the vastness.

I love the heart. It holds it all; it holds the love, the intimacy, the compassion, the forgiveness; and it holds the grief, the sorrow, the loss and all the pain you have endured and experienced since the moment you incarnated. The heart... the heart was the first thing that became YOU. The first thing that connected you to feeling. It knows all and it has its own "circuitry system." We spend our lives shielding and protecting our heart; we open it and then we close it. It gets damaged and it heals.

The heart is the true alchemist of our human-being because it can alchemize everything into love. Yes, that is correct. It can do this through the breath. Visualize the heart as you inhale, expanding exponentially and when you exhale, it empties completely. Every time you do that, imagine the heart and breath massaging what's in there, turning it into love. It will, if you allow it. If you open the heart and you surrender to its mystical possibility, it works magic.

What stops alchemy? Our mind. The illusions that we know it all. That we know better. The obligations, the responsibilities, the patterns and projections all stop the magic.

This is why I love yoga so much although I didn't know that was why until recently. It's the movement of the body in sync with the breath; it's the stillness of the mind amidst the busyness; it's the radical transformation that can happen when we are open and drop into the magic of the heart.

I say try it, what have you got to lose?

Cry, Laugh, Repeat

As I move into this new life of mine... the one that has always been there waiting for me to embrace it, I walk the line of presence while peeking at the past and moving into the future. I want to just put it all behind me and move into what is real for me now. However, I understand the importance of sharing... it is a gift and provides continual healing. And, from what I can see and have witnessed, if we are still here on this planet, navigating this human experience, we are still learning.

So I share.

I was numb in my marriage, going through the motions so I could "make it through the day." But it wasn't always like that. We started off super happy and connected and in love. We had lots of sex, traveled, saw the world and had plans to make a difference. You see, we all have a plan for what we want, but our expectations sometimes get in the way of what is real. When we realize it's time to shift, it can immobilize us, plague us and make us literally ill. So, for a while, we hang on tightly for whatever reason. We fall into an irrational fear of being alone. We rage against our own inner light and heartbeat, and then one day we say, "Basta! Enough!"

At the end of the road there is pain, anger, grief, resentment and fear, all bottled up in the body that wants so badly to experience joy and love and intimacy. But it's been broken. It has compromised and bent over backwards. It was in a state of massive confusion for so many years, it is rattled to its very core.

When the reality sets in, we say the words, we walk away from our dream and we are left alone and vulnerable. We are left with nothing but our decision; emotions are high and it is rough and ugly to be honest. We feel burdened, yet free at the same time. It is surreal, really. We know we made the right decision, yet it is so scary. People are hurt... lines are drawn... there's no going back.

On one level, the body and the mind are excited because each has been held captive for so long in a jail that was self-imposed and built brick by brick by your own illusion of bliss. On another level, it's like being put in the spin cycle of the washing machine. Leaving a marriage, no matter how long it lasted, no matter if you had kids or not, is like living two lives. It's like dying but being born again all in the same moment.

So what happens? Oh my... this new soul seeks love, it seeks protection, it seeks another heart and body to join with to connect with and share stories. It seeks what it thought it was missing for so many years. It is so afraid of being alone after all those years of sharing an illusion of love and intimacy.

The problem is that there are just so many splinters from the last relationship, which was held so deep. We look for love outside of ourselves as salve for our wounds. We look for something to protect us in this naked, vulnerable place in which we have put ourselves.

We seek partners to fill something... anything that will take away the pain. Only to relive the same issues we experienced that were left unresolved in our last relationship.

We have sex thinking that will cure everything. That in those moments of touch and ecstasy, that we will feel whole again. Able to protect ourselves from the storm that slams against our very existence.

The only way to fully experience that love with which we seek is to be it to ourselves.

To make dinner for ourselves, to make love to ourselves, to know what it feels like to feel true love and touch.

The goal is to stand naked... alive and awake to what is real.

Let me tell you... it means feeling gratitude for it all... not just the fun stuff but the hard shit... the yelling, the infidelity, the children, the trips, the divorce itself.

I think we toss the word *gratitude* around sometimes a bit carelessly.

Have gratitude for it all. What does that really mean anyway?

- Moving past the feeling that you are going to throw up when you think about the life you tossed away.

- Having no regret, and I mean *no* regret.

- Being happy when your ex has found someone else.

- Looking at your children, if you have them, and understanding that maybe they were the only reason you two were together... to birth these souls onto this planet.

- Loving and saying loving things when you drop down on the floor.

Why... because the world needs more love now... especially in times and relationships that are hard.

Because it feels better to love than it does to not love.

Don't toss yourself into something else right away; you have much to work out. You just whirled around in a life with someone who you most likely became one with.

Who are you now? Without that person?

Can you look at yourself in the mirror and love someone new?

Heal your body... heal your mind, heal your heart... for real.

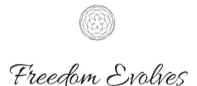

Freedom Evolves

I wrote about freedom a few years ago when I busted out of my old life and ran to my new one. Funny how the same topics come up over and over again and how we redefine them at various points of our life.

One truth... many expressions. Our truth expands and shifts along with our life, and if we hold fast to our beliefs at any one point in time, we really miss out. That's not say our values don't stay the same. I think they do. However... our truth about various beliefs we hold inevitably shift because, well, we are shifting.

So, this freedom thing. I had a conversation with a beautiful friend of mine the other day and we discussed this concept. She's made choices that have brought her an amazing husband, a two-year-old, a dog, and a stay-at-home job. Yet she feels trapped.

So I had to ask... what does freedom mean to you? For me, at eighteen it meant moving out of the house and into my own space where I could create, come home when I wanted, eat what I wanted and basically live the life I wanted.

When I got married my life shifted a bit because well, I think you do, to some degree, compromise your wants for the other person in that relationship. At least in the first marriage, anyway. I remember, before I got married or pregnant, I thought that my life was going to be this amazing travel-gypsy-nomadic existence. Filled with photography, a passport with thousands of stamps, friends all over the world, a backpack that held everything I needed and no one to answer to. To me, that was freedom.

So when I got married and realized that my husband had no desire to travel, I gave up that dream and found a compromise. I compromised because I thought that having that love meant more... I dragged him along to work on boats with me. That lasted for a while and we did have a great time, to be sure. No regrets.

He was compromising his freedom though, too, because his idea of freedom was working for a company that paid him well so he could play in his free time. So you see... our definition of freedom was different.

When I got pregnant I realized that my trip to Africa was out of the question. Not because I didn't think I could do it, but because, well, quite frankly I had made a life for myself that was already compromised. And without the support of my husband, we weren't going anywhere with this baby except to visit in-laws. And even that was a stretch.

At one point, I remember waking up from a dream where I was suffocating. Literally suffocating. I obviously did not feel free at all. I had no room to breathe. Freedom was something that I wanted in my heart but my choices over the years didn't really support that. And while I found deep love in my marriage and still find unexplainable gratitude for that phase in my life, my choices were not based on what I felt freedom to be.

So there I stood, suffocating and wondering how in the hell I was going to get out now that I had two (not one but two) kids, a dog, two cats, two mortgages, and a business. It was scary and overwhelming, to be honest. How could I have done this? All these shackles!

What I have come to learn from those experiences is that our choices in life are based on a moment in time. And on what we think we want in that moment. And when we shift and evolve and maybe even completely change through spirituality and study, our earlier choices look so messed up. In reality, they were divine.

And you needn't radically change your life either. You can change it two degrees and a powerful shift can happen from that. But sometimes it is like ripping a Band-Aid off. It hurts like hell.

But maybe if you just take a second and breathe into it you can find pockets of freedom in your life. Maybe when you breathe into those pockets and see the love through the mundane... then you really are experiencing freedom. You just don't know it because you have based your definition on something you made up at eighteen and how now you are thirty-five with a mortgage, two kids and a dog.

Hmmmm? What was your definition of freedom at eighteen? What is it now? I know when my kids were one and three it was going to Target with no one hanging on my leg! That was freedom. Now, at forty-five, it's being able to hang out with my two daughters and really listen to them. It's about writing from my heart and not being afraid of what people will think. It's about paying my own rent... doing yoga in my living room naked, playing with a partner who loves life as much as I do.

Knowing that I am me... in all forms in all moments and finding freedom where ever I am.

Look at your life now, now that maybe you have created roots. Notice and be mindful of your words here. Roots, not chains.

So freedom... what did it mean to you at eighteen? At twenty-five? At thirty-five? As a parent?

What did freedom mean to you between ages twenty and thirty?

What is it now?

How can you redefine it so you feel free in pockets... ?

Spirit... guide me today to my highest power... through word and deed give me the clarity necessary to live from a place that integrates truth, freedom and love.

Allow me to see the soul of every person who crosses my path today.

Allow me to see within the depths of my own soul, past the patterns that keep me in my ego.

Allow me to let love in courageously and fully and cease to block what is is naturally my birthright.

Help me to release patterns that keep me from experiencing my most divine manifestations of thought and joy.

Integrity

I wrote this blog at night and then completely changed it the next morning as the ultimate test of my own integrity came into play... as the themes always do.

It started off like this:

God, I love this word. I love it because it really does mean a lot to me. When I started looking at all the relationships I have in my life, the one thing that kept coming up for me was integrity. Integrity is so important. So I had to ask myself, why? Why is it so important? Why am I holding this word so dear to my heart?

When I looked it up online, it said:

> *the quality of being honest and having strong moral principles; moral uprightness.*

And this one said:

> *the state of being whole and undivided.*

Alright, well maybe I can get behind the state of being whole and undivided. But, from what? From whom? And what does "honest" or "strong moral principles" mean anyway? Isn't that a judgment call? Who says who has strong moral principles anyway? Who's in charge?

I personally like my definition better:

> *The state of being when your thoughts, words and deeds are in alignment with your soul's highest purpose and potential.*

That's a huge statement, I know. However, I do believe it to be true. And it got me thinking... okay, if that's true, how often are we really in integrity? I mean, really? How many times do we fall out of integrity with our deeds, our words or even our thoughts? Because you have to look at your thoughts too... it's starts there.

I've been witness to many people just in this yoga community, out of integrity. So much so that it makes me laugh! I've been witness to some of my own thoughts and I've had to say, "Wow... really? How can I think that? So not in my realm of being!" It doesn't happen often, but it does happen.

And in that moment, when I fall out of integrity, instead of judging myself and saying, "Oh shit, I must not be a yogi, I just had a impure thought!", I breathe and say, "Hmm, where did that thought come from?"

Because that is the work. Noticing when you fall out of integrity and then finding your way back in, and quickly. We all fall out of integrity and, let me tell you, if you think you don't, think again. That one act, that one word, that one thought; that's all it takes.

And then I had a moment where my own integrity was in question. And it wasn't about anything I was outwardly doing that was in question. No, in fact, it was how I was compromising my own integrity and standards for my own self, for my soul. It was an issue with how I was allowing myself to be treated, which was less than I deserved.

You see, I have always had an issue with wanting to make everyone happy. Always wanting peace and connection to prevail. Wanting a community that sings together, plays together, and hangs out together. And I always found that in the yoga community regardless of any city I live in or travel to. The yoga community is, hands down, the place to land no matter what; it's my tribe for sure.

This move to California has proven time and again to be the right decision. However, I must admit finally, that I personally have been tested on my commitment to integrity to my own soul. I allowed things to happen in my own life, compromised my ideals, and neglected my personal boundaries for the sake of making it happen in my life. For the promise of feeding my kids, finding a suitable home, and getting ourselves in a place that was safe, secure and lovely to come "home" to.

Yes, I did that, and I know I am not the only one that has.

You do that when you're a parent I think. You give up a part of yourself for the sake of what you think is important. And I did just that. I allowed myself to be treated in a way that was less than my soul deserved and I did it for a long time because the fulfillment I received from the yoga community more than made up for anything I was "giving away." I always felt loved and connected to every single person who walked my yoga classes and made connection with me.

But giving even a smidgen away of yourself, your ideals, and what you think you deserve will always come back to haunt you. And it has, and I can no longer allow it or hold space for it.

So then I started thinking about the fact that we are all doing this. All of us! And we're not trying to be mean or vindictive; we are just being human. So if we are all doing it, wouldn't it be nice if we all just kinda held some space for each other to be human?

I mean, I enjoy living the perfectly imperfect life. It keeps me off the hook and I get to tend to my own "side of the street" instead of worrying about what everyone else is doing.

For whatever reason, we all fall out of integrity. We all think a nasty thought, say something that's not so nice, and perhaps act in a way that is not in alignment with our soul. All of us!

So, now what? Take a breath, smirk or smile, and try not to judge your-self, but do explore the why behind that momentary shift in consciousness. Because it's a trigger for you to go deeper, to discover the root of why you would fall out of integrity. There's a deeper meaning, so explore that. And then notice it the next time it happens—because it will—and just do your best to do it differently next time.

And then remember, everyone else is trying to play this game of Life, so hold some space would ya?

My reason for falling out of integrity was fear. Of not being enough. Of not being able to make it on my own. Of not being accepted as I was... weird isn't it, the games our minds play?

So I say this... I hold no judgment, no remorse, no regret, no guilt and no resentment... Only deep, deep gratitude for:

The opportunity

The community

The connection

The courage

This life

The lessons

This tribe

But mostly, I am grateful for the exploration into the why. Because what I learned is that I am enough, I am doing it on my own and I am acceptable to myself just as I am, in this moment. Just as I am.

Karmic Action

I was having a discussion with some epic yogis the other day about karma and what defines karma yoga. We were talking about how karma yoga can be something as simple as being nice to people you don't know—picking up trash that's not yours or buying coffee for the person in line behind you without them knowing. That sort of "pay it forward" attitude.

While I love this idea, I still couldn't sit with karma just being a "do-gooder." It got me thinking a lot about karma and what it really means. I had to ask, first off, when you "do" that right action, what's your thought behind it? Are you doing it to get noticed? To make sure your karmic debt is in the green? Are you doing it because you want people to think you are a yogi? What's your reasoning behind this karmic action? Is there one?

When you "do" something for someone else, it needs to be for no reason at all. It needs to be... just to be. That is all. Is there is any agenda or wanting from this action? If so, it is not karmic action. Rather, it is ego intention.

Honestly, it's not even your actions that start the whole ball of karma wax moving. It is actually your thoughts. When you think a thought, immediately the transmitters in your brain speak to your chakras and you can feel expanded or contracted in one thought and one breath. So it all starts with your thoughts, and your thoughts never lie. Ever. How you choose to act on and manifest those thoughts is a much bigger topic.

But the main thing to remember is: You are karmically creating your path just with your thoughts. It is not just what you do; it is what you are thinking. Truly. So what are you thinking? Is it aligned with your actions? Make sure... because if not, there could be a bit of a mixup in what messages you are sending to the Universe.

And then another thought came to me:

Your karma is not just something you pay forward in order to be in right action; it is also the integrity with which you clean up what is behind you.

And I completely believe this.

I'm not sure if our "negative karmic debt" negates the positive "paying it forward" random acts of kindness. However, I do know that there is a balance between the two that has to happen. AND I believe it is happening in more moments than we realize.

Noticing those piles of unresolved business is the first step in cleaning up your karma. The second step is recognizing it as your "work" that will always be there.

As long as we are alive, we have karma.

We come in with it; we leave with it. Hopefully, we leave with less than we came in with but, again, that's another story. It does not really matter how many coffees you buy for the people behind you. What does matter is, how clean is your side of the street when you get in line to get those coffees?

One bit of insight as you move through your karmic action, intention, and debt. Tune into compassion along this journey—with yourself, that is. If we really do create our life with our thoughts, a lot of those thoughts are unconscious. But when we awaken to that knowledge as well as the accepting of our "debt," our only job is to clean up our karma with love, grace and responsibility.

Pain, Light and Love

It's amazing to me... this life, this body we walk around in, our thoughts, our dreams. This entire existence we call life. I slept through a good portion of mine, mainly because I was in pain and didn't really know how to deal with it. I had no tools at all! I kept running into pain and, after falling down over and over again, I began to numb, to stuff and ignore my pain. Traversing through life above my pain was my coping mechanism. Putting it away for another time was easier.

As a child we know that we are naturally connected to all that is. We know that we are naturally joyful. We know that we are one with the Universe. But sometimes we are born to families who have become hard and have forgotten that magical piece.

It's not their fault, it's an old pattern, one that I am at the forefront of, with many others, breaking through. I know differently, and thank God I know enough in time to share this important knowledge with my kids! That is what's most important, our lovely future generation. Still so pristine and awake. What a gift.

But pain is interesting to me. I believe that all physical pain is a manifestation of something deeper. Even accidents, I believe, can be caused by something deeper. Some unknown fear or imbalance in the emotional body. And what we do with that pain is indicative of how we are living our life.

My suggestion? Look at the pain deeply. What part of the body are you experiencing it in? How did it happen? Remember that you are a dense piece of matter with a soul. Look deeper into the pain. Don't just put a Band-Aid on it or take some pill to relieve the immediate annoyance. It's going to come back later and will keep coming back until you dig in and get to the root. The root is where the healing is. It's not in the surface scrape; it's deeper.

When I started studying the systems of the body and then the subtle body and then dove into the energy and ethereal, I began to remember. I remembered who I was beneath the pain: a really bright light. A being connected to God and to everything else that existed.

When you wake up to that, your life expands and it's amazing. You see everything differently! Life makes sense! You meet people just like you! And you all share and love and rejoice! Everything seems lighter!

However, if there is lingering pain, which there most likely is, you're still going to have to deal with it. But now you have tools and new friends, and you can practice looking at everything with compassion and grace. You can see your hurt from a new place that is blessed with forgiveness.

Pain is going to show up in your life over and over again. My invitation to you, and to us all, is to look at and examine it. See it for what it is and heal it, with every tool in your box.

I ask my girls, when I see them in pain, "Where are you feeling this? What does it feel like? Why do you think you're feeling it?" When they cry, they cry until they are done. When they are mad, they are mad until they are done. They have a safe place to share their feelings, no matter what. We are respectful; no outbursts in public places unless it HAS to happen. Let's try and wait until we at least get in the car, then we drop everything and listen.

They also know the energy body: the masculine and feminine and the chakras. They know enough to ask questions. These are the programs running everything as they have been forever. This knowledge is essential in healing the body on the root level.

I'm not sure all of our systems and chakras and life will ever be in perfect balance. However, I strive for learning, for expanding and growing every time something comes up. And I intend to share what I know, all my imperfections and works in progress, with these two little beings who are staring at me and listening to my every word.

I intend to remind them of what perfect beings they are amidst any bit of pain or trauma they may experience. That's what will expand ALL of our lives... that one bit of knowledge. Remember who you are... light and love.

Sovereignty

Sovereignty: *having supreme authority over oneself.* From a very young age, we tend to look outside ourselves for validation, guidance and information. I witness this every day with my two daughters. And as a parent, I know it's okay to validate and respond with praise but, at the same time, it's just as important if not MORE important, to allow them to make their own decisions (even though I'm cringing inside), so they can learn to gain that sense of sovereignty.

Turning to outside sources is pertinent for learning, growing and expanding. However, the end result will always be the same, and that is that growth is an inside job.

This can be quite scary if you have any smidgen of self-doubt, fear of failure, or decision-making issues. I've experienced all three, to be quite honest, and obtaining that sense of sovereignty has been quite a journey.

Self-sustaining action can be intimidating because, when we empower ourselves from the inside out, we truly have no one else to "blame" when things go unlike we planned. Not only that, but we also have to take complete ownership and responsibility for our thoughts, words and actions.

I'll repeat that: Complete ownership of our thoughts, words and actions.

That means that whatever we decide to be, do and contribute in this lifetime is ours to claim... regardless of how it turns out. But what I'm learning is... when we rely on the inner calling of our soul; we blaze our own trail and magnetize others that uplift our goals.

So then, can we confidently say that when we sit in meditation or dedication, and expand our innocence and vulnerability to learning for the sole purpose of elevating our soul's calling that we connect to our inner pulse and experience sovereignty?

Can we admit then that our external gaze actually inhibits our personal growth and may even restrict our intellect when it comes to making autonomous choices?

Would you agree then that relying on the projections (not the opinions), of others, can potentially take us down a path that is not our own?

I think that listening to the whisper of our own divinity and following that unique voice is the only way to gain the empowerment that we crave in this lifetime. I think we know on a deep level that we hold this power within ourselves to create what is uniquely ours, we just rely on the judgment of others and that then becomes the pattern.

Sovereignty is knowing your truth, standing in your truth and then expressing your truth in everything you do. Not just some of the time, all of the time.

Spiritual Ninja

You know, I have been asked so many times, "How in the world do you do it all? I mean, really: teaching in your community, raising two kids, managing your career, keeping up with your health... how?" I don't have a personal assistant, business manager or even a regular babysitter. Ha! That makes me laugh!

Truth be told: *I don't do it all*. I don't... I can't! No one can. Sometimes, I fall asleep while my little one reads to me. I leave dishes in the sink. Clothes live in the laundry basket and my furniture gets dusty. It happens! We try to stay organized and all have taken responsibility for their own "stuff," but sometimes connecting over a book or swimming in the pool is much more important.

I make choices in the moment as to what feels best, and I try to evaluate the consequences of my choices, but that doesn't often turn out as I anticipated, either. So I just do my best... that's it!

And, you know, I love my life. I'm so in love with it all that I don't really want to give up one thing. Not one! I get to live my passions every single day. I get to connect with hundreds of amazing people every single day. I get to listen to my girls' drama and sit IN it, every single day. I get to put together music and flows and share them with anyone who wants to play with me. I am living in one of the most beautiful places in the United States. We eat well, play well and have met the most generous, loving people along our path. Blessed life, to be sure.

I have zero complaints. Do I want more? Sometimes I would like to manifest about three more hours in my day so I could have lunch with a girlfriend, sneak away with my partner, or get a massage.

Our life is abundant, so abundant that things do slip through the cracks. Just the other night, as we prepared for the last day of school, I realized that I was going to miss my older daughter's poetry reading so I could take my little one to Angel Island on a field trip. My heart dropped... literally.

I didn't want to diminish the special time I would spend with my youngest and her friend, AND I wanted to be sure my oldest knew how much her event meant to me. Someone was going to feel left out.

Over the last year, I have let go of the need to "feel bad," though. I don't feel bad... I don't have time to feel bad! I think, as long as we express our love in other ways, all the time, no one will EVER feel left out. In fact, they may even support one another, which is what I found to be a new truth that I welcome in gladly!

I do have a few secrets in getting to the other side of guilt and allowing oneself to receive, and I'm happy to share. You needn't have kids to use these, either... these are just good living tips.

- Don't try to do it all. Understand that you are going to miss something. You are going to have to choose... you can't possibly do it all. So if you are one of those people trying... stop it right now.

- Hang out with other people who get it. Why? Because you will be able to help each other. I couldn't do anything without this amazing group of parents that I hang out with. (As I write this, I'm receiving a video text from a mom who recorded my daughter reading her poetry. And I'm crying in a public place. My kids would be so embarrassed.)

- Don't take anything personally. I mean it. Nothing is about you, nothing. Stop wasting your time in that thought process.

- Make time for yourself... what fills you up? For me, it's yoga, dance and being in nature—specifically near the ocean. Do what fills you up, even if you steal fleeting moments.

- Optimal self-care is key. I don't mean go to the gym every single day; I mean optimal, deep self-care. Take a walk, engage in a spiritual practice that is sacred, sit and read, eat nourishing food, limit or eliminate alcohol and sugar, sleep... yes, sleep.

- Be particular with your relationships. Don't try to be everything to everybody; your space is sacred. Do YOU first, your family next, and then draw in those individuals that fill you up. When you are filled, it's easy to give.

- Receive the help... receive the support... receive the love... This might be a tough one for you, but you must do it. When you receive you are telling the Universe that you do not want to control anything AND that you are worthy of this gift. Take it and say thank you.

It's tiring, trying to do it all. The feminine energy that is moving and flowing everywhere is begging for a softness to take over. I don't know about you but I grew up learning the complete opposite. The unlearning that can be challenging, but you can do it.

Thank God, this is a process, a practice. And thank God, I get to get up and do it all over again, every single day.

Best part of my day? Listening to two nine-year-olds giggle in the backseat while eating chocolate croissants; hearing them laugh at the ferry all the way down the street; finding a new coffee shop to work at that overlooks the bay; watching a video of my daughter recite her poem; and sitting in gratitude for my lovely friends.

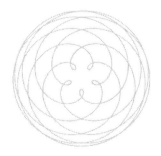

Truth—Freedom—Love

I have this tattoo on my right arm, my inner arm. It's there to remind me every day of what I believe to be true. And that is this:

When we live in truth, deep, resounding truth, we liberate ourselves from the illusions that we created based on old patterns and beliefs. And, in that process, we are then able to experience deep, authentic love within ourselves, which illuminates love in everything.

This has been a hard lesson for me to learn, as it is for several thousand people, I am sure. We are easily influenced by our parents' ideas, riddled with ancestral patterns, persuaded by society, and scared of our inner light. Add a dose of ego and need for recognition, and we can almost guarantee ourselves a life that is mediocre or with regret.

I decided to tattoo this on my arm so that every single time I entered *Adho Muka Svasana*, countless times a week, I would remember.

- I would remember when I wasn't fully in my integrity.

- I would notice when my ego was running the show.

- I would remember when I made a choice that was less than my highest good.

- I would notice when I wasn't honoring both the light and the dark sides of myself.

Living life consciously sometimes feel like a dance of two steps forward, one step back. Doing that dance with compassion and humor is key, because life is all about practicing and, if we're still here, we have work to do. Moving into deep truth is the work, and it's not always easy.

Just beyond that fear of peering over the edge and taking that leap: That is where the magic lives. As humans, we are conditioned to avoid pain, escape change and even mask our truth, especially if it doesn't fit into the "box" of society.

Know your truth and live it every day:

1. Turn off the news. It is riddled with negativity, and if you want to fully step into your truth, you've got to turn off the outside noise.

2. Sit with yourself and make a list of what you love, what you are good at, what people love about you, and what scares the hell out of you.

3. Recognize your fear in moving forward; this is your deepest work. This is the jewel of your soul. Breathe into it and become enamored by it. It is the bridge that you will cross many times to continually propel you forward.

4. Pain is an initiation of up-leveling your vibration. Notice it, embrace it, and transmute it to courage.

5. Be open to others of like mind and heart walking this path. They are going to arrive in droves, trust me.

6. Develop compassion for yourself as you step out on this new path.

7. Notice any resistance to this shift and dive deeper into inquiry around that resistance.

8. Be open to detours and challenges because those experiences are your biggest lessons.

9. Stay laser focused on your path. It is your unique soul imprint; someone else's will never fulfill you.

Understand that you are consistently and forever evolving. Your core values stay the same but your truth may shift and change. We are consistently being asked to live more authentically and up-level our vibration so we can live our highest truth. If you are still here, there is work to do. And everything that happens in your life happens to give you the courage to show up more fully in that purpose.

Be ready for it all—a simple right turn or a radical shift in perspective and direction. You are here to evolve, share and heal. Keep focusing inward on you and the rest will take care of itself.

CHAPTER 6

Intuition and New Beginnings
Ajna Chakra

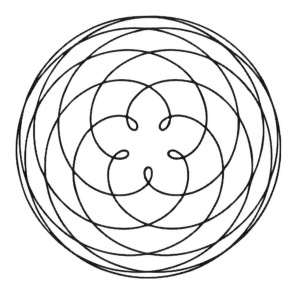

Crystal Clarity

This essay was written in October 2014, two years after moving from the Northwest to San Francisco. I had dropped everything to relocate myself and my children. Started my yoga business over again. Fast forward just one year, to November 2015: every single one of the items listed as intentions for 2015 was completed. Always, in awe and reverence for our power to create.

I'm sitting here doing my schedule for the next three to six months and I realize again, how fortunate I am.

The last four years have been a whirlwind while I gather myself up and "realign and redesign" my life. It's such a wonderful place to be, in this life—contributing, dancing, working, laughing and BEing.

I've been DOing a lot these past few years; admittedly some choices have come out of fear and/or survival mode. That chapter, now completely over, I am supported, confident, and crystal clear about how I feel in just about every moment I am engaged in. Not only that, but my intuition is on high alert, pointing me in every direction I need to go.

I asked students today to use the words "crystal clarity" as their focus for the week. Why not just clarity? Why crystal clarity? Because now is the time for complete focus in what it is that you are passionate about so you can DO THAT instead of distracting yourself with anything else.

We find that crystal clarity by truly tapping into what feels good and what does not. We trust that the Universe has our back and that everything happening to us is actually happening for us. We let go of all victimization and stand in our stories, ready to witness the revelation. We fall into tempo with the Universe and everything rearranges without a ton of effort or struggle.

Dial in the aperture on the lens of your life. You can no longer live out of focus. The world needs people ready and willing to use this life and

LOVE this life. Ground into your feet and ask to be clear. When you are in a moment, feel into that space between the belly and the heart.

Feel into **that** space in any exchange, any decision, any relationship you are experiencing. It's your beacon of truth and it will tell you: Expand or contract.

Then ground into that truth and open your eyes wide to see the clarity of it all. Trust in the truth. It may be totally different than what you are experiencing right now or it might be spot on. Just know it and begin to embody it... all the way. Not just half-assed.

Here's my clarity:

Over the next few months I am participating in a training to lead girls and their mothers on an amazing journey of self-discovery and expansion. I am also learning about astrology and yoga and how the two combined bring us closer to the rhythms of the planets. Not only that, but I will finish my Reiki certification as well as go back to using essential oils in my classes and my work.

All of this in preparation for 2015, when I launch my 200- and 300-hour yoga teacher training and the revolutionary Girls Elevate. The lens of my life has come into clear focus and seemingly everything else is falling away.

Now I ask you... what are you clear about? What is your passion? Sit... breathe... ask.

Divine Guidance

The theme started out as *trust*, which is such an epic word. But I wanted to go deeper than trust. Deeper than intellectual thought. Deeper than what we think we know to be true.

The word trust provokes emotion in some people, namely me. Divine guidance on the other hand, *makes me feel like I'm only part human and mostly fairy dust.* Which on some days is much easier than being human.

But I think that this human experience is only challenging if we make it so. I think the problems and dramas arise when we don't listen to that Divine guidance. When we instead barrel forward with a sense of profound know-it-all speed.

From what I have found, and this is from my experience anyway, Divine guidance is like a nice hammock that holds you suspended in space. You know you're safe and contained, and you can see things from a higher perspective because what's coming to you is from a higher perspective that your brain can't possibly create.

A lot of times, I find people shutting their Divine guidance down with rational thoughts, obligatory responses, and ancestral patterns, closing themselves off to the magic of being guided. I believe that fear of listening to this guidance comes from thinking that they know it all. Or maybe it's just too damn comfortable, this default reality, that they can't possibly entertain any kind of shift from a mysterious voice, thought, or dream.

Because, honestly, and I can say this from experience, Divine guidance isn't always an obvious stroll in the park that is actually horse drawn, in a heated cart, with some gorgeous man (or woman) feeding you grapes along the way. It's not always a simple path from A to B that offers you complete grace and ease and a promise of gold chocolates at the end. But it can be!

But mostly, Divine guidance is asking you to "please move in a direction that is more in alignment with your soul." And, sometimes, it begins as a whisper in your ear but can escalate to drama in your life, forcing you to shift in some way. And some of you may still fight it, which is always interesting.

And I think that Divine guidance is really something like an oasis of miracles. It's like a pool of lotus flowers that have messages in them. It's the ONLY way to do things. And please note, that I'm all about intellectual reasoning, creating spreadsheets and budgets, timelines and all that masculine manifesting stuff. That piece has to happen in order for anything to exist. However... I believe and function by the reality of Divine guidance... every single day.

I think that some people fear it and others, like myself, thrive in it. It drives some people crazy when I say that I have to really drop into the situation before I can make a decision. But you know, that's how I do it. And trust me, it has not always been neat and tidy, these musings from my Internal Guidance System (IGS). But apparently I was way off course for some odd reason. The turbulence definitely diminished once I started to listen.

And I also think that depending upon how far you have shifted off course by not listening to it along the way will be directly proportional to how loud, disruptive and annoying the shift will be. I say, try not to fight it, listen and then trust it.

Divine guidance, yeah. Believe it or not, there is a force out there that knows more than you do, witnesses things from a higher perspective than you do, understands your karma more than you do, and is trying, so lovingly, to help you. I invite you to listen, act accordingly and—even if you have to squint your eyes and jump fearlessly—do it. It will be the best leap you ever took, listening to that voice.

From Darkness to Light

I've had thousands of New Year's wishes and anthems come into my awareness these last few days leading up to today. So many, it's almost overwhelming. This whole instant-access-to-information can be daunting and too much for one person to navigate, honestly.

There are a couple of things, though, that I have found important enough to share as we move into this New Year on this New Moon.

1. What are the three most powerful shifts that transformed you this past year—the ones that opened your heart to love?

When you sit and reflect on your life this past year, what brings a smile to your face and warmth to your heart that is palpable? What brings your breath to an exhale because that moment in time is so alive in your heart it fills you up the instant you think about it? Remember those times and hold them dear to your heart with gratitude and grace.

2. *What are the three most powerful shifts that transformed you this past year—the ones that rocked you to your core, shook the very essence of your being... and THEN opened your heart to love?*

Consider acknowledging those moments that hurt your heart so deeply you fell to your knees. Or scared you so badly, it took you a minute to catch your breath. You know the ones. The abandonment, the physical injury, the fear of losing something or someone, the grief, the guilt, the conflict... we all have those moments.

Take that same breath you had when you brought the loving, gracious moments into your awareness, and wash over these "not so perfect" moments with a deep exhalation of appreciation. It may take a minute, but do it anyway. Because guess what? In order to move forward truthfully, you must understand equanimity and have faith and trust in it all. It is all perfect. It really is.

3. *What does friendship mean to you?*

Friendships are important, and, to be very transparent, in my last three years of completely transforming my life, I have lost several friends. For some, it was time to let go. For others, however, it wasn't. But I was too focused on my stuff and didn't give them the nurturing space and love they needed to grow and trust and love our connection.

It's how life works sometimes, so we can't beat ourselves up. We can only move forward with what we know now, in this moment. So ask yourself, what does true friendship mean to you? And then BE that to your friends.

4. *How deep and potent are your connections?*

Listen, Facebook does NOT KNOW your *20 Most Powerful Moments of 2013*. Only you do. Your "Friends" on Facebook are not your friends. Well, maybe some of them are, and yes, it's nice to have loving energy thrown your way from your closest 1,000 buddies. However, at the end of the day, can you look your friends in the eye and tell them something difficult? Can you sit in silence and just listen when they speak about you and give you feedback? Have you opened your heart to love and intimacy? How truthful are you when someone says, "How are you?" Can you recognize another's love, pain, joy and connection?

Can you feel another's heart beat when you embrace them? How deeply are you willing to connect to your Self this coming year so you can deeply connect with another? Are you there for your friends as they are for you? What friendships are important to you? Are you being the friend you want them to be to you?

5. *What magic are you willing to create this coming year? Where can you dig deep and find courage?*

If you are your own powerful creator, and your thoughts create your life, what are you thinking right now? About other people? About yourself? Your worthiness? About the world in general, and where and how you stand in it? Are your thoughts positive, skewed, chaotic or deliberate? How are you thinking?

Streamline your thoughts and articulate them so you manifest your heart's desires this coming year. Allow yourself to be distracted because hello, you ARE human after all! But in the stillness of one breath, bring yourself back on track.

What have you been most afraid of?... Do that!

6. *What can you let go of gracefully and lovingly as you move forward?*

For any movement to happen, we must be willing to let go of something. It's a balance of energy. We can't keep filling up if we are already full. What are you willing to let go of, with love and appreciation for the purpose it served? A pattern? A thought? A person? What is it?

As we move from darkness to light and head into yet another year of our lives... take a moment today to sit in your accomplishments of the year. Find grace and gratitude for it all. Let it all fill your heart with joy and love. It's all important and necessary... all of it.

And as you move into this New Year, take the least amount of baggage from last year so you are free to feel truth, freedom and love.

Deep bows to all my teachers, every single one who has crossed my path and has shown me a reflection of who I am in that moment. Deep bows to my own imperfections. Deep bows to the compassion and love available in every single moment. May we all move from darkness to light and live with truth, compassion, gratitude, purpose, power and passion.

How to Love an Empath

When I was a kid, I felt like I was looking at my life through a magnifying glass. I could feel the energy around me so intensely. Innocently, I thought everyone was like that. When I mentioned this feeling to others, they labeled me as weird and different.

Maybe the word *empath* did not exist back then. What is an empath anyway? *A person with the paranormal ability to apprehend the mental or emotional state of another individual.* Not only that, but most of us are also highly intuitive and see things. Our dreams tell stories; we believe in fairies and we still witness magic on a daily basis. We know how you are feeling. We know the truth.

Time and again, when I would bring something up that I was feeling, I was told, "Oh no honey, that's not it at all. You really shouldn't feel that way." It was challenging, to see the truth of what was happening and to keep it to myself.

From that conditioning, I began to doubt myself and my abilities. It was easier to numb my feelings than to explore them. I would second-guess myself, keep quiet and say nothing. My swirling thoughts took over; I knew the truth but the outside world told me that I was wrong.

Call me crazy, but I am witnessing more and more of us empaths and intuitives speaking up out there... loudly. We know the Earth needs help; we see the burden on the next seven generations and we know that it is our responsibility to take action now. So we have to break out of our shell and go for it. It is pretty incredible.

Want to love an empath?

Make space for us to breathe and express. I admit, sometimes my feelings come out and make no sense at all. I have gotten better over the years but it is still radical to some. Open your heart while I am speaking my truth. It may take me a minute and I may have to circle back around a time or two, but I will get there.

For God's sake, **don't judge us or tell us to be quiet or not feel**. That would be a death sentence. Feeling is how we navigate our way through life, so telling us not to feel a certain way, or that our feelings are wrong is like kicking us in the shin.

Trust us. We may not have a mathematical equation that maps everything out, but we feel it. There may never be a rational reason why we make a decision, we just feel into it and we know it is right. That is just how we live our life.

When we break free from the plan and take a different road, don't get mad or upset; **enjoy the ride**. Eventually we may end up at the same place but maybe we won't. We just know that the divine plan is better than we could have imagined.

Listen to us... believe us when we say we have a crazy dream. Believe us when we say we see fairies! Believe us when we say anything. We don't live a lie... EVER... we live truth... ALL THE TIME.

Don't be afraid of us. We won't turn you into a frog. Just don't lie to us, okay? We can handle truth... that's the only way we can function. We are powerful, yes, but, at the same time, we really enjoy someone to lean on, cuddle with, laugh with and enjoy this beautiful life with.

Give us time to write, pray, meditate and be alone with our thoughts. We have to have peaceful quiet. When we walk away from you, it's not because we don't love you. We do. We just have to download for a little bit. It is very important for our work and our heart. Oh, and loud noises and big crowds give us the willies... it's too much energy and we cannot see or feel straight. We can take it in small doses, but not for too long.

Massage us with your hands, your words and your thoughts. We are raw and we like it that way. We don't do well when we have to shut down. And, we pick up other people's energy easily. So helping us to release that through massage, yoga, hiking in nature, holding hands, using kind words and loving thoughts really helps. We are affected by it all... truly.

As an empath, we are responsible to protect our energy, yes. But we also don't want to close off... it is not in our nature. So yes, we will do our part and practice "safe connection," but we still need help from those closest to us. The ones who see us. The ones who spend a lot of time with us. We need you the most.

And if you don't get it... just try. It's important and we love you.

I Believe

If you would have told me three years ago that this would be my life, I would have laughed in your face! You see, three years ago I was separating from my then husband, letting it all go, arguing over things like the house and the furniture. And now, I'm playing in Marin, San Francisco, Aspen, Portland and Tahoe! AND I'm home for my kids in the late afternoons.

What do I say to that? I say I BELIEVE.

It wasn't that long ago that I was in fear and desperation... it really wasn't. But at the same time, it feels like another lifetime ago. Even when I look at photos of myself, I am blown away at the difference, the clarity, the wisdom and the grace.

Here's the deal... and I'm going to keep this simple:

Your thoughts create your reality. And not only that, but your feelings and emotions behind those thoughts, play a huge part in creating your life. You see, your soul body knows when you don't believe in yourself. So if you say things like, "REALLY?" or, "I can't believe this is happening!" or, "What did I do to deserve this?"... you are basically tossing your gifts away.

You get in your own way... all the time! So wake up and believe.

Believe in what?

In love; in magic; in synchronicity; in life; in kindness; in healing; in forgiveness.

Not only CAN you create your life, you ARE creating your life. What are you creating exactly? Be clear... be committed... watch it formulate... it's happening!

It's time to get out of fear mode, let all your negative patterns drop and move forward in trust, intuition and grace.

Ready... Set... Go!!!!

Intuition

All week I have been playing in the realm of *intuitive guidance*. In fact, one of my phrases for the year is intuitive guidance. Being open to it, as always, but more than that, actually following it.

Really dropping in and listening... intently. Not questioning, not wondering, but actually following through.

I find that it's really easy to "drop in" when there isn't anything happening out of the ordinary, you know, like life! But you know, the reality is, life is always happening and it's really easy to get tossed off your game of connection if you're not paying attention!

There's all these various ways to tap into your intuition and each of us has a sense of what works. Here are a few:

Visionary experience. *You may use your third eye and literally vision things.*

Audio experience. *You may hear things, almost like whispers from the Divine. You can hear it in nature, in waves, wind and the birds.*

Feeling with entire body. *The truth is that we feel other people's energy all the time; the trick is to notice how you feel.*

Gut reaction. *You just know it in your gut or in your heart.*

Download from the crown chakra. *You experience guidance in a complete statement or sentence.*

Dream time. *Sometimes your intuition speaks in your dreams, mostly through symbolism.*

Personally, I use them all on various occasions and when I find them hard to locate—meaning I am scattered, confused or in my head—I get on my mat and plug in. Literally, I plug into the energy that vibrates with my every step. Tap into the energy that swirls around my head with messages of Divine love and guidance. Connect to the internal guidance system that can't wait to assist me in following my heart.

Intuition is something we feel; it's not something we do. It's a nudge, a push, an energy that, when cultivated, can guide us along our most divine path of Being. It's the synchronicity of events that link together to create a bigger picture of what is.

The problem is we aren't in our feeling body all that often. And we miss events that actually mean something. In fact, we spend more time in our head trying to figure things out. The ironic thing is, if we let go of the grip and allow the breadcrumbs to lead us along the path, all would flow in an intuitive way.

Here's a mantra for you: I amplify in stillness. Does that mean you have to sit still to amplify your awareness? Well, no, not really. Messages come in clearer if you do, for sure! But the intention is to find that connection in movement, in chaos, in discomfort... so you can move from a place that is guided and not reactionary.

It's a practice... a life-long practice. Don't rush, but please, start listening today. The time is now to get on your path and I'm thinking that if you don't, something is going to push you onto it, whether you like it or not.

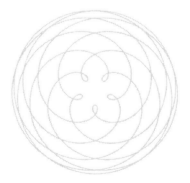

Lean Into It

What would it be like to lean back into what life is offering you and absorb it, accept it and become it? What would it feel like to fall into the flow of your life with trust and abandon?

This is a tough one for most of us because we think we know it all. We plan, we organize, we rationalize and we expect that life is going to go a certain way. And, to be honest, most of the time it doesn't quite go the way we plan. And in those instances our instinct is to fight it, to rebel, to struggle and to keep trying.

It's like putting a square peg into a round hole. It's never going to work. Well maybe it will, if we shave the sides off, round some edges and force it in... then it will work. But usually something gives and whatever it was we were struggling to be, do or create, implodes.

The other part of leaning back, which came to me like a lightening bolt this week, was leaning back into our community when we need support.

Truth: *You are supported... all the time.* So when you hear yourself say, "I can't do this," or "I'm in this all alone," or "No one understands me," you are dead wrong. That vibration just doesn't feel good because it's not truth.

This past week my daughter was really sick... still is. Out of nowhere came neighbors, friends, clients and colleagues offering up support. Your only job, when that happens, is to accept it. No, "I can't believe it!" or "I owe you!"... just receive the help and receive the love.

After a challenging week, I was grateful to lead hundreds of yogis through some fun postures and warming flow at Wanderlust in the City. We started off the session by putting our arms around strangers and holding them up from behind in support. Rows and rows of people supporting each other. I wanted them to feel what it felt like to truly lean back in trust of another. It was beautiful... powerful. Such an epic reminder.

Here's the deal, we are never alone, ever. This is how you do it: ask for help; realize your deservedness; receive it. Without question, just receive. Lean back and say thank you.

Yup that's how it works.

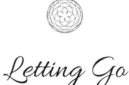

Letting Go

Letting go chose me this week. I was lying in bed Sunday morning wondering what the theme for the week would be. Racking my brain, thinking, thinking, thinking. We had had such a busy week and, honestly, my brain couldn't hold another drop of information.

My nine-year-old came in and cuddled up next to me and I said, "Ava, what shall we drum up for our theme this week?" It was the morning they were leaving for a week and flying to Portland to visit their dad over Thanksgiving. She lay there, not moving, looking up at the ceiling and said, "How about letting go, mommy?"

My heart skipped a beat, as it always does when she says something so profound and accurate. Of course it was letting go, of course it was.

I had been contemplating this concept as I always do at this time of the year. Not only were we still reeling in the New Moon energy, but we were also on the brink of a New Year. November has always been my time to re-evaluate anyway.

So *letting go* it was.

I started to think about what we are so tightly wound and attached to. And how much we wrap ourselves up in so many things: expectations, ideas, concepts, people, tradition and patterns, to toss out a few ideas, anyway. Then I fell upon our own identity.

"What do you do?" Oh, I'm a mother, an author, yoga teacher, student, ex-wife, coach, friend... name it. There are so many labels and roles we play as human BE-ings, aren't there? What would happen if we dropped just one? Or at the very least took a look at what no longer fulfills us and decided to let it go?

And, oh my, what would happen if we, for one day, allowed ourselves to NOT BE THAT? And just be nothing, with no label and no identity? What then?

You see, I think we have lots and lots of labels as we move through life. If we are wise, we allow ourselves many opportunities to "try on" identities and see how they fit. The key, though, is not to attach to them. Because, once we attach, we are inhibiting ourselves from the potential of a miracle. And at the bottom of those labels, what are we anyway?

Light, love, infinite energy, ever-changing...

Labels confine us. They keep us in something and limit our thinking, most often from the perspective of other people. However, when we drop those labels and allow ourselves to sit in our own greatness, the possibilities are endless.

I try always to go back to this: The brain is an amazing organ and can think and create in linear time. However, it cannot possibly conceive of the heart's magic. Because it can only know what it knows. Anything out of that realm is... seemingly inconceivable.

I don't know about you, but on most days, I like to play in the inconceivable. But... the thing is, you have to let go. And you can't let go for a REASON... or IN EXCHANGE for something else. You have to let go for the promise of NOTHING... for the inconceivable... for the miracle.

So yeah, you have to trust. You have to trust that beneath it all, you are an amazing, ever changing, ever evolving being of light, who has unlimited potential and an outrageous view on life.

Letting go is seemingly scary, but for once, if only for a moment, I invite you to let go of the labels. Drop them like a hot potato. Sit in the unknown, in the potential of nothing. Don't search for what comes up... just sit in the nothing. Breathe into its spaciousness... its vastness... its pulsating beat.

Just be there for a minute. There is everything in letting go, everything.

Need to Know

"You don't have to see the entire staircase, just take the first step," said a very wise man named Martin Luther King Jr. So very, very true.

But what do we do instead? We try to plan it all out. We look ahead in our life, not considering how valuable it would be if we looked within instead. We are asked to "map out" the next ten years of our life when we're just children. We're asked to commit to a job, relationship, home mortgage, and some other tangible thing, when we don't know if that is really what we want... or will want in ten years' time.

We have no idea who we are, where we came from, what makes us tick, what we love or what our passions are, yet we are asked to commit to a "goal."

We spend years and heaps of money going to college while taking no time at all exploring the depths of our souls. We compare ourselves to other things people have done, what other people have accomplished, and try and "get to" a point in our life that is... "something like that."

We are programmed from a very early age that we "need to know" what's next. We "need to know" what we want, how to get it, and when it will come. And, God forbid it doesn't come the way we want, how we planned, or wrapped up in a pretty little package. Then all hell breaks loose, or worse yet, we label ourselves as a failure.

This is ludicrous.

Over the past couple of years, I've been playing with the idea of letting go of the need to know. And I've been talking to a lot of people who are having issues with this need to know illness.

I've witnessed miracles in letting go, experienced joy in just BEing, and felt a sense of calm when I allowed the nothingness to take over. I'm a self-admitted Recovering Type A, which means I may never "get over" my need to know, I just catch myself much more quickly, now, and relax into the not knowing without fighting it.

I've been here before and I took a huge leap into the unknown a few years ago. Everything turned out just fine—actually, better than I could have imagined. And, to be honest, I've learned that if you actually adapt "not knowing" into your daily life, you may only need to make 2 to 5 degree turns in direction in order to stay on "course" instead of 180 degree leaps into an abyss.

The truth is, we have no idea what is next.

The truth is, our brain is so friggin' small in comparison to the Universe. How on Earth do we think that we can even THINK we know what's next? And HOW to get there? And that we have control?

Are you flippin' kidding me?

So I say, we stop with the whole need to know and just be for a hot little minute. I'm not saying that we shouldn't plan, or think, or intend, or manifest. What I am saying, though, is that we should allow for the magic of the unknown to take hold and send us somewhere totally unplanned. That we should allow for our paths to be altered and shifted according to the Universal plan instead of our pea-sized brain.

Here's the deal: The brain works in patterns; the Universe works in magical spirals for which there are no formulas. Magic spirals sound way more fun, don't'cha think?

Not Knowing

Happy Solstice, lovely...

In this tipping point, at the pinnacle of light and dark, may you celebrate in wonderment all the transformations taking place in your life right now. May you look at the road behind you with satisfaction, respect and gratitude. May you look at the road ahead, perhaps not knowing exactly where you're going, but heading forward with trust, devotion, and love.

Can you pay attention to what is falling from your life, and what is magnetizing—creating momentum and excitement? May you have the courage to drop what is not working, knowing that it will make the space necessary for something magical to show up gently and lovingly.

As I mentioned, this last Mercury retrograde did a number on me. As I look at what I currently "do" on this planet, I am reminded, again, about the importance of discernment and clarity. I will never claim to know it all, but I do know that things in my life need a bit more organizing.

What that looks like, I'm not quite sure, but I'm going to start somewhere and I'm going to start with the passing of the New Moon, the start of Summer Solstice and the theme of Not Knowing. Yeah... pretty much spot on.

How we present ourselves to the world is an important key to manifesting the life we desire. And while I love all that I get to "do," I also value "being," which I haven't been experiencing a whole lot of lately.

I have a problem. And I think it's a problem that a lot of people have. It's the "I need to know" syndrome. Have you heard of it? It could show up like this:

I need to know what's next.

I need to know how much that costs.

I need to know what the weather is like.

I need to know where my kids are.

I need to know what to do when I arrive at my destination.

I need to know what my past lover is doing.

I need to know what is happening on Facebook, Twitter and Instagram.

You feel me?

I would like to publicly admit that I may never, ever eradicate the need to know. Mainly because, well, there are some things that I really do need to know.

I can honestly say that after this trip to Tulum, I remembered that I don't really need to know much. And, not only that, but what I do know will most likely shift. And some of what I know is a lie or an illusion anyway. And, most importantly, in the not knowing, there is space for magic, creation, and miracles.

In the not knowing, the Now can occur. The magic of the Now can usher you toward something unexpected. The not planning actually makes way for mystical encounters. And, the not knowing offers an oasis of unimaginable experiences and undeniable clarity.

In the space of not knowing we release control.

In the space of not knowing we allow spirit to come through and whoosh us away.

In the space of not knowing we say, Thy will... not My will.

I'm not saying I will never "need to know" again. What I am saying is that I am committed to being in the not knowing a lot more. Starting right now.

I experienced a hurricane upon arriving to Tulum, a barrier in the language, a chance meeting of a dear friend, reflections of my old self, glimpses and dreams of my new self, a miraculous raw food hut, waves crashing at my window to lull me to sleep, yoga every day, sitting in the womb of the Mother Earth, and an amazing sense of clarity.

Say yes to not knowing and allow the unknown to infiltrate your being. In the not knowing and the not planning, truth bubbles to the surface so eloquently that you can't help but breathe it in and allow it to whisk you away.

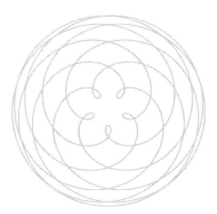

Rebirth

When we think of a rebirth we think of starting over, and that is very true. Also true, we are rebirthing ourselves in many moments, consciously or unconsciously because we are always shifting. Always. We are not sedentary people. We change all the time because we are subject to so many ideas of how to do things, see things and experience things. At the touch of a screen you are given an opportunity to shift your reality. Truth.

Rebirthing can be epic, life changing and traumatic.

This entire week has been synchronicity after synchronicity, and you know what theme kept coming up, wherever I turned? Rebirth.

It's no mistake that my new friend Katy Komenda wrote about the lag time of the full moon and how we are rebirthing ourselves. It's not happenstance that I had the opportunity to listen to an amazing recording with Sally Kempton and Andrew Harvey talking about the Evolutionary Goddess. Who did they talk about? The Goddess Kali, not in the sense of who she "is," but how she is showing up on this planet right now. And, it's no coincidence that my dear teacher Elayne Kalila Doughty drummed in the Goddess Kali for all of us priestesses to experience Kali live in our circle and in our dreams for days after.

It's Kali and she's here—the creator, the destroyer and the preserver. And she's over it already. She's over the lies and the illusions with how we have been living. She's destroying everything we thought we knew, and she's done playing around. She arrives angry and obliterates anything that is even a half-truth. Frankly, she could care less what you think or what excuse you have.

You see, her gift is that she sees what is on the other side. She sees the jewels in the midst and she just doesn't have the patience to wait around for you to figure it out! She demolishes out of love and deep compassion, but it doesn't always seem that way.

We have to put up with this rant and rage to get to the other side, though. You see, on the other side is a version of life, your life, that your pea-sized brain—in comparison to the Universe—could never conceive of. She knows all and she loves all. She just has a way about getting you to comply; she knows you need a rebirth and she's pushing you out the door already!

You know what part I love about Kali the most, though? Her ability to preserve and to see the jewel in the midst of chaos and destruction. When the smoke and ash are clearing... when the Earth stops shaking, quaking, melting, drought-ing and whatever other natural disaster she creates comes to an end, she is there, walking through the rubble to remind us of the jewel beneath it all.

This is rebirthing. Knowing there is a jewel, a uniqueness, a gift within you that EVERYONE on this planet can see—and that for some of you, is waiting to be expressed. Rebirthing is allowing an aspect of you to die in order to truly see what is real about YOU.

Receptivity

You open the heart, you say YES. But, then, why do your dreams not manifest? Why then are you still overwhelmed? Why are you still working so hard to figure it all out? Why are you still searching? Why are you still wallowing in the drama? Paying attention to the small stuff? Allowing others' ideas to influence your thoughts and actions? Why do you continue allowing the outside stuff to create your life? How long can you continue to miss the big picture... the destiny that you mapped out for yourself before you signed up for this life on Earth? How much longer are you going to allow that to be your story? When are you really going to show up as your Self with a capital S?

What is it going to take?

For most, it takes a kick in the rear by the Universe. A material world loss or an attachment taken away... these usually push people to new heights of awareness. But only after one crawls out from under the rubble of pain, anguish and victimization of that loss.

Sounds like a lot of energy spent if you ask me. What if it really was easier than that? What if it really was as easy as living from your heart, listening intently and then having faith?

Randomly, I reread a blog on clarity and decided to take the theme of clarity very seriously. I went home and created a sacred space with a special altar; I committed to a daily meditation practice every morning and every evening. I became very aware of my energy and how I was using it—manifesting powerful teachers who could further that learning for me. I found breath in every single, stressful moment. I paused before I spoke. I looked people in the eyes when they talked to me. I turned off the alerts on my phone. I shut my eyes to sleep—on most nights anyway—by 10 p.m.

I asked... "How can I serve? Point me to my path." I didn't ask how... I just said ok. I said, "Allow me to hear the voice of intuition above all else. Let me say yes without fear." I paid attention to the outside world, but only as if it were a movie made just for me. And guess what? Clarity came. Profound clarity. Ear ringing, angel singing, goosebump-rising clarity.

And all along the way, the "signs," the "omens," the "coincidences" were never questioned. They were welcomed with gratitude. I never once turned away from the Universe saying things like, "I can't BELIEVE this is happening!" Or questioning by proclaiming, "REALLY? I'm not sure I can handle this. This is too much for me." Or "I can't do that!"

I believed that each moment was a sign... each moment was a gift. Even the ones when I was called out on my lack of presence, patience, authenticity and judgment. I welcomed each moment and showed up with vulnerability and unconditional love for myself and for the person or situation. I detached completely from what I thought I knew and gave in to what IS.

Where is this going?

To receptivity: being completely open to what shows up, for REAL this time, with NO conditions. It's a gift to live from your heart; loving so deeply you can feel your heart vibrating and swelling to its most expanded expression. It's an even greater gift to see, with laser-sharp intensity and clarity, your path, your vision, your destiny. So, now... there it is... now what?

Plan? Ask how?

No, breathe it in... give thanks... allow the Universe, allow God to give it to you. Give it space to breathe and come to you fully. Allow the pieces of the puzzle to present themselves in their Divine time. You will know the EXACT moment it's time to move into that space. You will know EXACTLY what to do when it is time. Every single thing you need will be given to you, as if by magic.

I'm ready... are you?

Resonance

Resonance, as defined by Webster is, *the reinforcement or prolongation of sound by reflection from a surface or by the synchronous vibration of a neighboring object.*

That is the physics definition.

I love that.

What's interesting to me is that we ARE a vibrating field. The field starts at our heart. That's the pulse, the spanda, that starts it all, and then we vibrate outward from there. AND everyone else you encounter is also a vibrating field. AND not only that but every living thing has its own vibrating field. AND if that's not enough, Mother Earth has Her own vibrating field that starts at her core as well.

So here we all are, vibrating around each other. And, the amazing thing is, we get to decide what we want to vibrate with and who we want to become resonant with. Now I know that's hard to visualize because there is so much happening in one moment, isn't there? I mean, really, we take in more information in a minute than we will ever use. And more information in a day comes to us than people experienced in their entire lives only a century ago.

Welcome to the age of efficient, technical connection.

We multi-task and get caught up in other people's stuff so easily and realize we aren't resonant at all with what's happening in that moment. The static of our mind gets so loud that it becomes hard to hear what the vibration of the heart is actually saying... which, by the way, is... your truth.

We must stop multi-tasking, stop splitting our attention and drop into empty presence with one thing. Yes, *one* thing. And it's not our thought, judgment or emotion around that instant... it's just that instant we drop into with breath.

When you stop doing multiple things at one time, you become present to one thing and everything else drops away. This, according to physics, actually allows more things with that same vibration to come to you and other things to drop away. Everything comes into support of that one thing you are focusing on. It's profound.

And we can train our mind to be in one moment at a time by breathing into empty presence with what is and focusing on one thing at a time. In doing so, all the support, love, connection and resonance you will ever need falls to you without a struggle.

We want to be that still-point, walk in stillness, and connect with oneness as often as possible so we can hear the heart over everything else. When we hear the heart, the noise, the chaos, the distractions and the static all drop away.

Train yourself to be in your higher field of awareness by focusing on one thing at a time. Multi-tasking brings us into the chaos, confuses the mind and skews our internal compass. Do one thing at a time and you will feel resonance with what is Truth.

Space

The girls and I moved into a new home this past weekend that offers us so much more space. People would come over and say, "Wow, look at all this space!" And I found myself, in those moments, wanting to justify and explain, *why the space*. As if we didn't deserve it, or something. I continually go to the root of things though... that's just who I am. So I had to think about it for a moment. What did I do when I was given more space to create, breathe, share and love?

Apparently, I felt like I didn't deserve it.

So this made me look at what we do when we have space.

Space is infinite but somehow, we try to quantify it. We try to measure it and claim it. But, the reality is, it is infinite and always changing and adjusting to our life.

Meaning when you "have" more space, it is because you need that space to grow, contemplate, expand or share it with someone else. You don't "have" any more space; the Universe is just offering you more because, well, you need it.

So with that in mind, I started thinking about what we do with space when we "get" it. Do we fill it up right away? Do we justify having it? Do we immediately put things in it? And what about when there is space in a conversation? Do we talk just to talk? And space in a relationship? Or in our day? Do we "do" something to... "do" something?

What would happen if we just sat in the space and were grateful for it? Really looked at it as a gift? Gave it the time it needs to transmute into what it wants to create? What if we were still and quiet and just sat in it? What if, when there was space in a relationship, we could just allow that space to expand our awareness of what is real? If we could look at ourselves and how we are relating—take a moment to inquire what we're actually doing?

I think it would make a difference and here's why:

In space there is infinite breath. There is nothing and everything all at once. In space lives the Divine, and although she is whispering to us all the time, it is in space that she gets to speak the loudest. Space is a gift from the Universe that offers expansion into our idea of time, our awareness, and our connection with the Divine and all that is.

So in those moments, what do you do?

It's easy to recognize space in your body when you're on your mat. It's easy to notice space between thought and reaction. It's easy to notice the space when you take long deep breaths.

So what do you do in those moments?

Here's what I do:

I pause, sit still and take note of my emotions and where I'm feeling whatever I'm feeling.

I resist the urge to talk, do something or fill it up.

I consider what I am meant to witness, notice or understand in this moment.

I listen intently.

I let my kids slide around the house in their socks before I go buying a bunch of furniture that I'm going to have to dust.

Here's the deal. Space is infinite and cannot be measured, quantified, created or destroyed. We all "take up" space, we share our space, we give away our space, we allow people into our space, and we protect our space.

A great practice is to observe what you do with yours. Is it creating expansion in your life or constriction? Are you distracted, addicted or confused in your space? Or do you tap into the Divine and download what is being offered?

The choice is totally yours and you get to decide. Just remember that it is a gift. Like the breath, it is gift. And like breath, you can choose how deep and expansive you want to go.

Trust

I'm writing this as I sit in a hotel room in Denver, not really sure about how I got here. Don't get me wrong, I know how I got to this hotel, just not really sure about how I got to this moment. I'm here to promote my non-profit Girls Elevate; I'm here to connect with a new community; I'm here to film some online yoga videos; and I'm here to catch a breath.

I feel so fortunate to live the life I do and, at the same time, I know I created it. I don't say that from an ego standpoint, it's just a fact. I have always lived a life that has been a bit... on the edge or different from the norm, if you will.

And every time I have made a change, or done things a little differently, it required huge amounts of trust in myself. To be perfectly transparent, that has not always been easy because self-doubt and worthiness is my deal, my work.

However, beyond the wavering trust I have and have not had in myself, I have always had a trust in Universal support. So, for example, I have always known that no matter how things are "going," it's perfectly divine.

I moved from Michigan to San Diego when I was twenty-one—no job, just did it. It was an epic choice! I took off for the South Pacific and Australia for an indefinite amount of time after I graduated college, life changing. I came back to San Diego—a bit linear for me but all worked out well. Moved to Florida and traveled a huge part of the world on a yacht as a chef. Can I say... BEST DECISION EVER!

Moved to the Northwest with a one-year-old. Everything worked out perfectly, especially the cleansing rain. Created lots of clarity for me. Decided to really change my life and sold my business, got divorced, and moved to San Francisco all in one year... crazy brave but I trusted and... I would say I'm sitting pretty nice.

Now... trust doesn't mean lucky. It doesn't mean easy. It means trusting. Trusting in the unknown... in your own abilities... in those voices that tell you... YES... NOW!!!! Saying... okay and... not really knowing what you're doing.

Like today... I was trying to leave San Francisco and get to the airport on time and for some odd reason, my GPS just stops working. I pulled over and talked on the phone for about fifteen minutes with Verizon until they fixed it... no explanation for this "quirky mishap," the guy said.

The Universe kept me safe from something. No idea what it was; it doesn't matter.

Silly things like this keep me believing.

I never worry about anything, really... at least I try not to. If we sit still enough and we listen intently, we are being guided all the time. If we ask for help, it comes. And if we listen to our heart, it will always show us the way. But only 100 percent of the time.

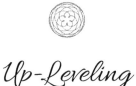

Up-Leveling

We are offered countless opportunities to up-level our vibration on any given day. And this does NOT mean:

We are perfect;

We are better than anyone else; or

We have achieved something in our life.

No. Actually, up-leveling means that we are now more aware.

More aware of our thoughts, our actions, our words and more aware of how we function in the world. We are more aware of how we show up in relationship, what we want in life and how to get there. We look outside ourselves and witness the reality and truth of what IS.

Up-leveling gets you nowhere in particular but more awake. And, if you're doing it "right," you are always offered the opportunity to up-level; whether or not you take that opportunity is entirely up to you.

Up-leveling your vibration is not all that easy. It's actually quite challenging because it requires letting go of old stuff and moving into what you may LABEL as unfamiliar. It's actually easier to get snagged by limiting beliefs, old patterns, and the lower vibration of other people in your path than it is to raise your own vibration. Now with social media, it's so easy to get distracted by all the publicly announced accomplishments of everyone else than it is to focus on your own stuff. Raising your vibration requires work; there's no doubt about it.

I was laughing this week because, well, this theme so resonates with me right now. I was sitting there, going through my task list for the week and amidst the "blog post, social media training/posts, enter emails, update site" was "prepare for meeting with Dove, get processes outlined for assistant, send grant proposal to Lululemon, prepare for meeting with potential business manager, read through proposal from book publisher."

But wait... then, on my other sticky note pile, there was, "reformat computer, take photos off phone, update and back up phone, complete relocation order for children, and get summer schedule for kids together." Needless to say, I went to Juice Alley, decided to juice this week, and ran up and down the Lyon Street steps all week long just to clear my head and heart.

That is up-leveling—having a lot happening at one time and being able to see above it. Noticing the "balls in the air" and recognizing how each one is integral to the other. Becoming extremely aware that something is shifting, noticing that this may have been offered before, but this time, you will do something different to support the elevation. And in all this shifting, you get a bit uncomfortable but you do it anyway. Because in that uncomfortable space, something does shift. It's a release of old patterns; it's a letting go of old beliefs, and it's a trust that this time will be different because you are different. We up-level our energy when we:

Look at the stillness and locate our distractions;

Recognize what is holding us back and sit in the un-comfortableness;

Take care of old "business" or "karma" that weighs us down;

Acknowledge our greatness and move toward it; and

Embrace the truth that we deserve all the amazingness coming our way.

Up-leveling, sharing our gifts, learning, growing, letting go and shining anew, is why we're here.

Renew --- rethink --- realign --- reignite --- rewire

Shift everything you think you know into an up-leveled version, which means, you may think you do not know what you're doing, but on some level, I promise you do. And when you leave the familiarity with no promise of something bigger or better... you will fall into a flow that is so familiar, you won't remember what it was like before.

CHAPTER 7

Astral Energy
Sahasrara Chakra

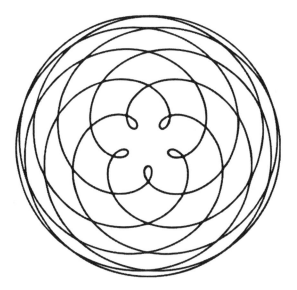

Balance

Thank Goddess for this theme! After all the astrological upheaval that began all the way back with Venus retrograde, followed by a deep dive into the Sun by Venus, followed by a Solar eclipse, then Mercury in retrograde, then a Lunar eclipse, finishing with Mercury stationing direct, where else can we go but into balance?

During this time that began in August (before Burning Man for me, personally, and, I'm sure, for others at that gathering), I've been witness to a huge cleanse, epic transformations, upheavals, intense realizations, and brave leaps forward by so many. And for me personally, well, let's just say that there have been radical shifts that would put an earthquake to shame.

There are many places I'm sure we could go after all that, but really, we must choose balance.

Let me say that again: We must choose balance. I say that deliberately because it is your choice and you know that; I know you do.

When I reviewed the astrological orchestra and then realized (as if it could be any other way), that Navratri began just after the New Moon, I literally dropped to my knees and gave thanks.

Let me start here:

This New Moon in Libra is all about balance—specifically, balance in relationships. And, in case you forgot, you have relationships all over the place: with others, with your past, with your parents, with your job, with yourself, with money, with the Earth, and even with your choices. Name it; you're in relationship all the time. And this New Moon is asking you to bring into balance what has been off "karmic kilter" for quite some time. All that shakedown that came before this moment, what was that all about? It's all been preparing you for this moment.

The one where truth resides, where compassion lives, where abundance is obvious, where love wins, and where you exhale and listen to your intuitive knowing—feeling that deep resonance with all that is.

Sounds very prophetic, doesn't it? Well, it's true.

Now, follow me here; let me take this to the next step:

For a moment, think about all the people on this planet now celebrating Navratri, the worship of the Divine Feminine in all her forms. They are praying, fasting, celebrating, chanting, yoga-ing, talking about and—maybe for the first time—recognizing the radiance of the Divine Feminine. They are receiving the energy of the Great Mother by bowing to her greatness. So, even if none of this resonates with you personally, it's happening, and it's powerful beyond your thinking mind.

Trust me on this one, please.

The truth is that our world has been out of balance for a very, very long time. The story, as it is told in many traditions and lineages, has been about patriarchal rule and how it has created our now seemingly insurmountable issues.

I personally love the story about Shiva and Sati and how she promises to marry Shiva and help create the World, but only if she is always honored and respected for her power. The moment the "powers that be" forget who she is and disregard her power and try to take over, she leaves her body. Shiva is pissed off and begins careening through the world with her broken physical form, spewing obscenities. Everywhere he goes, major earth tragedies begin happening.

Saturn comes in and begins dropping pieces of Sati's body to the Earth in the hopes of stopping Shiva from complete destruction. According to this story, which I love, where Sati's body landed, we now experience major vortexes, magical geography, and deep connection with the Divine Feminine—because this is where She resides.

So I ask you now... how has that changed from whatever lineage you believe in, whatever text you want to read from? How has that changed? Have we not been overruled by old, out dated, patriarchal ideals and concepts? Has the feminine not been disrespected, undervalued, and in many cases, manipulated for some type of consumption or greed?

The answer is yes, yes, it has. And the time to stop is now. The time is now to make changes. Big or small, it doesn't matter, just make a change.

Now.

Admittedly, change is happening and it is happening at a pretty quick rate, which makes me so happy. I see it mostly in amazing, vulnerable, authentic, available men who recognize the beauty of the Divine and are excited to talk about it. I see it in women coming together in circle and supporting each other. I see it in an overall sense of receiving... allowing... accepting... unconditional loving.

And now, in this moment, the planets, the stars, the Moon, and the energy of the Divine Feminine herself are asking us to please find balance. And to please do it now.

To some, that sounds and feels overwhelming. I mean, with all the "issues" we are currently experiencing, how can one person possibly bring anything into balance? It's seemingly too much.

Now let me take you here:

What if you could, for a moment, believe in the truth of a holographic Universe? Meaning that every single thing you were experiencing and witnessing was a mere reflection of yourself and how you "relate" in the world. What if that were true?

Which it is.

Then can you maybe just take a moment in silence and truly recognize the truth of what is imbalance in your own life? Can you really look at the dark shadows of your life and admit that you have the power to create balance for yourself? See and begin to shift the ways in which you push and force, and disallow love, harmony, spirit to create FOR you?

Can you sit in receptivity for a hot minute and drink in the beauty of what is occurring? Can you welcome the idea that change is necessary and that maybe we needn't be doing so much and maybe we should be okay with receiving? And heart knowing? And intuitive guidance?

That's what it's going to take—a swift turn to the heart to experience this balance. By all of us. Together as one.

How... you ask? Well, first off, we needn't ever ask how. But if you need something, a checklist of sorts... Here you go:

Sit

Breathe

Revel in nature

Say yes

Listen

Love... unapologetically

Forgive... and mean it

BE the energy of the Divine

Honor Her...

Honor your mother, your wife, your daughter, and honor the feminine that resides in every single man on this planet. Because guess what? From what I'm hearing... a lot of them are wanting to shift, but they are so damn afraid of disappointing us. They know... on a deep level, they know, that we are the Shakti of creation. And they too, have been emasculated by our own imbalance of masculine energy.

There's no manual on how to do this differently! They can only go into the heart where many of them, and the ones before them, have never even traveled—where many of them were hurt and told to fight, and consume, and gain, and win instead of love.

Support them with your loving grace. Hold them in times of transformation. And love them for trying.

This is where balance will happen. In your home. In the way you love. In the way you receive. In the way you acknowledge all phases of the Divine within yourself.

Your fierce compassion *(Durga)*

Your infinite generosity *(Lakshmi)*

Your intuitive guidance *(Saraswati)*

This practice is more than postures sequenced together to create a class. This is about moving your body in time with the rhythm of the Universe. And it's happening... with or without you, it's happening.

Change of Seasons

I will never claim to know it all... I don't want to know it all.

However, I have been studying how the yoga experience can be enhanced (that is, bring you closer to yourself), by using essential oils and crystals, chanting, and looking up at the stars every now and again. Call me a witchy woman if you want, but it works. And I know it works because when I look in the mirror I say, "Ah, there I am!"

In class, I have been talking a lot about letting go, setting intentions, and really getting clear about what you want to be, do and contribute on this planet. This is no joke, guys. I mean, what I KNOW to be true is this: When you state it... it comes! And lately it's been very swift.

I can honestly say that although I don't know everything, I do know that a change of seasons outside ourselves usually ignites a change of season inside ourselves. And everything in this moment is saying, "Hang on sister, there's a storm coming!"

Before you gasp, know that storms aren't always torrential or "bad." Although every now and again I want to say, "Really? I thought I just weathered one! Aren't we done yet?"

No, we are not done, because we are still here. Therefore, we will continue to weather storms, go through transition, morph, grow and change. And as far as I am concerned, as a collective, we really benefit from a nice storm to shake things up.

We have to be ready.

With any change of season, I ask you:

What do you want to be, do and contribute on this planet? Because the Universe is not joking around. Mother Earth needs you and your gifts, so it is time. I think it has always been "time"... there are just a lot of us waking up is all, and the planet is excited to get things rolling!

Now being in tune with this season, I ask you an even more important question:

What have you found to be expanding for you thus far? What can you honor and acknowledge in this past season that has now brought you to right here, right now? Because the reality is that you created everything that is happening in your life with your thoughts and it is showing up as your present moment. What are you grateful for right now? Can you look at your ancestral lineage and find some gratitude for those folks too? Because they have had a hand in your amazingness to be sure.

Autumn Equinox is the time of the year when the daylight and sunlight are equal to each other. It is a time of harvest, of going in, or honoring what you have done thus far, finding gratitude, and taking a much needed rest as the days get darker. It's time to contemplate and be prepared for the next season when you will plant your seeds.

You want to be sure you are planting a garden that will fulfill your needs, desires, and dharma, right?

So get clear... really clear. Sit and observe. Contemplate. Get quiet. Stop talking so much and listen in on your heartbeat. You've done enough now... it is time to rest.

Dream Big

"You are ending a recent and significant underground-type of journey, but the good news is that it ends with Friday's solar eclipse/new moon. Above ground you go! Much like a coal miner coming out of the cave they work in, the light looks brighter—shockingly so—when we emerge. The air smells fresher. The sounds sing sweeter." These are the words of my astrologer about my Leo path. I'm not sure she realizes just how spot on she is with this.

You see...

About six years before this post, I had decided to leave a life that was seemingly so stable and lovely and secure. From the outside it was beautiful and perfect. But inside I knew I was dying. And as I look back from an even deeper place, I know now, there wasn't anything wrong with my life; I just wasn't being true to myself. I had hidden myself behind so much and I knew I couldn't shine until I faced it all.

I knew I had to leave, but there was so much preparation that had to happen. I slipped into an underground survival mode and went to work. I stashed money away, worked my ass off, and prayed every day. I prayed for forgiveness, for clarity, for protection, for grace, and for truth. But most of all, for freedom.

Freedom from my pain, my past, my hurt and the lies I told myself about what my life was supposed to be. I had put myself in a safe little box, but my light was not shining... at least I didn't feel it. People around me could see it. But my heart was so, it was so clouded by my past, I just couldn't see it. And I didn't feel safe to share it completely. There was healing to be done and it could not happen in the space I was in.

I knew I had to leave in 2009 but spent an entire year planning and praying. Then, in 2010 I traveled to Squaw Valley with two very dear friends and on our way back to the Northwest, I told them I would be leaving my current life. I was gifted a beautiful bracelet that said DREAM BIG. I wore it every single day for four years until it broke.

In 2011 my life completely unraveled and I was scared shitless. The noise outside of my head was so loud and it was an effort to block it out, listening to only my heart. I realized this underground journey had only just begun. Through fear, guilt, shame, rage, grief, judgment, ridicule and projection, I kept walking, kept yoga-ing, kept praying, and kept diving in deep.

Only 11 months into the first transition, in 2012 I was offered an opportunity to change my life even more and I took it. It would change things drastically and force me to step out onto a huge ledge...

You are going to be alone in this.

You must be self-sustaining.

You must leave your two daughters for a little bit of time.

It was heart-wrenching and still brings tears to my eyes, thinking about it. But the BIG DREAM required BIG RISK. And keep in mind, big risk is just that, it's a risk; there are no guarantees. And let me be clear; the BIG DREAM had nothing to do with fame or fortune... only freedom.

Truth, freedom and love. Period.

My relocation to California wasn't all roses and chocolate. Nope. It involved being vulnerable, open, hard work, and sleeping on lots of couches. It involved asking for help and kicking ass. It involved me looking at all of my dark stuff with truth and compassion. It involved setting boundaries that hurt and put me into a space of even more needed isolation. It involved losing my mind over my heart, big time. It involved leaving my soulmate whom I loved dearly. It involved crying alone and meditating a lot. It meant putting lots of miles on my car in the hopes of making a difference and an impact.

You see, when you leave it all and arrive with only what fits in your car, you start over. You believe, you trust, and you keep loving. You keep praying, you keep yoga-ing, and you keep moving. There isn't time for intimacy, or partnership, or doubting, or partying. There is work to be done when you rebuild for the sake of a big dream.

In 2013 my lovely daughters moved back in with me. After nine months of being apart, nine months of traveling into the dark corners of my life, nine months of deep introspection, I emerged a lighter being. My heart was at ease. But still, there was work to be done, as always. Still somewhat underground.

My dream... truth, freedom and love. Period.

In 2014 I could afford to take my kids to Palm Desert on vacation. I stopped worrying about how I was going to pay for food. I could finally breathe a bit easier and didn't grind my teeth at night. I stopped fighting about what I thought was fair or right and began falling into the space of flow instead.

2014 felt good. I dreamed big. I saw my light and moved swiftly into an even brighter light, which of course is scary, but so necessary.

Truth, freedom and love. Period.

For two and a half years, we lived in an apartment that was on the bottom floor of our building and faced the trees. We didn't get direct light, but it was beautiful. I remembering purchasing a little furniture set for our small back deck. My kids did their homework out there and argued over who can use the table.

Every time I walked up those three flights of steps, I emerged from the beauty of my safe place, my apartment where I became self-sustaining, self-loving and at ease with growing. The words that permeate my heart when I emerge every single morning are:

"I am so ready to move up into the light."

It's time to dream bigger than you can imagine. Don't plan it, just move into the light without fear, doubt or worry. It's time.

And within one year of writing this blog, my children and I moved into a beautiful home where they each have their own bedroom and I have my own bathroom. We have a large backyard with a deck, garden boxes and room to run. Our back window overlooks Mt. Tamalpais and inside is full of love, life and connection. We moved into the light.

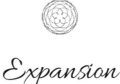

Expansion

Wow! We are being asked to expand big time.

Do you feel it? Are you feeling pulled? Constricted? Weepy? Have you emotionally vomited for no apparent reason? Felt like you're being ushered into a new reality?

That's because you are. Whether you know it or not, whether you are accepting of it or not, whether you want to or not, you are. And it's getting real.

We are just days away from this super full moon lunar eclipse and it's big. I mean, big. It's being called the astrological event of the year. Of the year! I've had a hard time talking in class this week, the energy is so palpable for me. Not only that, but that full moon is going to be eclipsed on Sunday night. It's crazy and wonderful and needed and pushing every single button for some of us.

It's asking us to look at whatever has been swept under the rug, ignored, covered up and pushed to the side. It's asking us to toss out all the old because room for the new must be made. Jupiter is asking us to expand our container; for some of us... in every area of our lives. And this is so uncomfortable isn't it? Moving into a new reality that is big and expansive and bright. I mean, sometimes it is uncomfortable to sit in your greatness, isn't it?

But why is that? What the heck? Oh the ego...

Not only that, but Saturn is now in Sagittarius and, from what I hear, until about 2017. And if you remember, Sagittarius is the energy that says GO... DO IT! It's the fire in our lives that burns like crazy if we let it. But Saturn likes organization. So the goal now is to move, move now and... again after the dust has settled. Create a thoughtful process and strategic plan that will allow your life to unfold into divine action without any more running on the "hamster wheel."

I liken this to a "controlled burn." So eloquently served to me. Thank you, Petra.

My suggestion: Sit in it. Sit in all of it; the full moon, the magnification, the truth, the fear, the discomfort, the fire, the ego. Sit in the eclipse on Sunday night and then allow those moments of darkness to wash over you like an astrological bath of lifetimes. Cleansing you from all the old paradigm stuff that keeps you from this current reality of... .

EXPANSION

I get it, okay? I totally do. My life is expanding in ways that I cannot even begin to explain. Every phase of my life is opening up. And at the gateway of every door, I meet fear. I meet this old friend who says, "Are you sure? Are you sure you are are ready for this? Have you considered your attachments? Your ethics? Your doubts? Have you looked at all of it deeply enough? Because if you have... GO. And if you haven't, then go ahead and sit with me some more because we could do this for year. For lifetimes! I have nothing else to do but harass you if that's what you want."

At least that is what my fear tells me. I have decided to make friends with my fear. Let me tell you, it's been the best friendship thus far.

I have dreamt about this expansion, meditated on it, felt it in my body and envisioned the beauty that is coming; the magic that has always been there. I always feel energy in my arm; my arms have always been my conduit and they have been so active this week. I can't get enough Chataurangas and inversions, to be honest.

So I do it.

I keep expanding, keep allowing, keep courageously loving my fears because beyond that is flippin' magic. I've felt it. I have felt the realm beyond this human body I walk around in every day.

Have you? Have you expanded your breath just enough to remember that you are more than this human experience? If not... start right now. It's not too late.

Super easy... breathe. Expand. Breathe. Expand. Breathe. Expand.

Keep hitting the repeat button and do nothing else. Let this epic, magical, astrological show compliment—not dictate... compliment your ever-expanding awareness into what is real. And let go of the rest.

If you remember anything at all, remember this. You are this epically incarnated human being that is full of fairy dust. At any point in time you have the choice to get caught up in the noise, haste and contraction of the drama that comes along with being human. But... the beauty of that is you also have the choice to step back, as far back as the edge of your reality, and see how small things really are. It is there that you see just how expansive you really are.

Trust me.

Magic

I totally believe in magic. I do. There is no explanation for every single thing on this planet; there just isn't. Although, if you think there is, I am open to hearing your answers. I bet you will be exhausted by the time you finish, though.

Not believing in magic means you have an "equation" that works out every single time, for every single thing. It also means that you can control everything about everything and that it's all black and white.

I don't know... there seems to be something wrong with that.

I'm living in vibrant color these days, and it's flippin' magical! I say things and they appear, give or take a day or two. I feel something, and it manifests. I have to be really, really careful with my thoughts these days. Truth!

Here's the deal that brought me to magic...

The stars, the planets, the cosmos, none of us know exactly how they got here, right? I mean for sure, for sure. You don't know, right? If you do, please tell me! Do you have it on video?

And, we don't get to control the way they all move up there in the Universe, as far as I'm aware. And, what about the whole "energy of the Moon"? I mean, it creates the waves on the Earth! That's kinda crazy, isn't it?

And how about your own body? You know, the one you walk around in all day, every day? Do you wake up and turn your systems on and make sure everything is working according to your plan? No, I didn't think so. It just does its thing. Even while you're sleeping!

I'm mesmerized by that!

I still remember looking at my daughter, at 2:00 a.m. when she was five days old. She was crying and crying, screaming really. And I held her on my lap and looked down her throat and thought, "Wow, I grew that in my belly." Astounding.

That's magic.

Our body and how it moves, and how the brain functions... to me, magic. And I know doctors have scientific answers for everything, but I say, yeah, whatever. There has to be some magic in there somewhere. You can't know it all, you just cannot!

And what about synchronicity? Or unexpected events? What about love? Have you ever met your soulmate? Or your twin flame? Have you ever met someone and instantly felt connected to them, like you had met them before? Or had such chemistry the moment you laid eyes on them? Have you ever been so connected to your dreams that you woke up and that dream manifested within a day, a week, a month?

I think our society discounts magic too much. We think too much and rationalize too much and put things in categories and label everything so it "makes sense." Magic doesn't make sense. It just is and it just happens.

We can't plan everything... you don't WANT to plan everything! At least I don't.

I want to take care of what I need to take care of, make sure my bills get paid, my kids get where they need to get to (which is magic on some days) and skillfully continue to find passion in my "work" until the day I pass.

In between all of that, I am open to the magic of it all. I am open to looking into my lover's eyes and knowing our meeting was magic. I'm open to staring at the ocean and contemplating all its majestic unknown rhythms. I am open to not knowing if any Hindu or Greek mythology story is true or not. And I'm open to loving the magic of life unfolding before my eyes.

It's way more fun that way, don't cha think?

Navarati

Life is funny, isn't it? I mean, we have all these dimensions to ourselves and sometimes live in all of them at the same time. I laugh out loud when I realize I'm in two or three dimensions at once. This can be both enlightening and horrifying depending on who I am hanging out with at the moment.

Another chuckle for me this past week: the new moon in Libra, coupled with the Autumn equinox, now THAT's funny! AND did you know that there is a lunar eclipse on October 8? Followed by the full moon on October 17? Suffice it to say, there is a lot happening out there, which means there may be a lot happening inside as well.

We must be present to it if we want to stay in the game and remain grounded while life (and the planets) whirl around us.

So, this brings me back to life being funny. The other day, at the new moon, I am on the phone with a dear friend of mine, and he says, "You know it's Navarati tomorrow, right?" And I gasp and say, "I totally forgot!" Why did I forget? Because I didn't put it on my Google calendar, that's why! Because it didn't fall into the "volleyball/soccer schedule." Because it was also Rosh Hashanah and my kids had the day off school, which I also forgot about so... yes, this slipped my bandwidth.

So, I'm up late, reading about Navarati, listening to Sally Kempton, looking around my house that I just HAD to organize because it felt necessary. And I'm also answering emails from over two weeks ago, and I'm laughing. Laughing because it all makes me wonder how I do it!

Because the question that keeps coming up is, how in the heck do you integrate this goddess energy when there are so many other things happening in our external human experience? I mean, really, I'm writing this while my younger daughter videotapes herself on her new "cooking show," and my older daughter does her hair for volleyball practice. (And by doing her hair, I mean she's putting hot pink streaks in it!)

Oh, and there is chicken marinating in the sink and laundry going two buildings down. Thank God homework is done.

REALLY????? Goddess energy? Calling it in? How? When???? How do you do THAT amidst all the humanity out there!

Thankfully, I KNOW that connecting with this Goddess/Divine Feminine energy is important. It's all I think about, really, and it's not about ME, it's about it all. Everything can be related to the ha-tha on this planet. The balance and Divine order of this very planet rests on our own ability to find that ha-tha within ourselves. And I have to admit, there are days I feel like I fall short. But, mostly, I believe that I am enough.

I remember every day that I am a "house-holder." I am not a monk or a goddess, high on a mountaintop with nothing to do but chant and meditate all day. No, my life is much more abundant than that, and not only that, but being a householder, doing my best to embody goddess energy, IS my work right now. The devotion I have to my children is strong and steady, and that is where I find my true goddess power.

What about me, you ask? How do I get my Lakshmi on? When do I call on Lakshmi? How do I know what I need? How do I stay out of the chaos and drop into my heart immediately?

Here are some tips:

- Every single morning, okay, maybe every other morning, sit for a minimum of five minutes and breathe. Ask the Divine to guide you. Just ask for guidance and presence in your day.

- Keep your space organized and cleaned up from clutter. Make it happy and light. Use candles, flowers, incense... anything that you define as beautiful and bountiful.

- Make space in your calendar for you... you needn't explain, justify or reason about what that is, just do it with no excuses. Ask for help if necessary.

- Hang out in nature. Commune with the trees, the mountain, the beach, the sand... sit in it. Put your hands on it, feel it and embody it all. Stand in awe of Mother Gaia at least once a day.

- When someone does something nice for you, don't ask why, don't question it and don't think you have to "pay them back." Say, "I receive that, thank you." And accept it.

Listen, I get it. We are all doing our thing moving around this planet, making things happen, connecting, creating and DOing.

Goddess energy is about BEing and ALLowing and REceiving. Let's do that.

My commitment during Navarati?

Digital detox... Doing what I can to disconnect with DISCONNECTION on the last day of Navarati.

Green juice every morning, red juice at night.

Walking after dinner with my kids or SITTING in the grass during soccer practice.

Reading from my new book, *Wild Creative* by Tami Lyn Kent, every single evening before bed.

What's yours? Share it, do it, integrate it.

New Moon Energy

You know, my life has always followed this crazy rhythm. And it hasn't always been in time with everyone else's. However, what I'm learning is that it has been in Divine time and, very often, in time with the Moon.

This Mercury retrograde did a number on me, for sure. I felt like I was on the Tilt-a-Wheel these last three weeks; remember that flippin' ride? When I was a kid, I hated that ride but now, as an adult, I thrive on it.

Over the last three weeks I was asked, by the Universe, to up-level. And that meant to drop the things that weren't working, re-evaluate the things that were causing some angst, get some support, go out on a limb, pay more attention to my kids, incorporate self-care back into my routine, and take a hot minute to just sit down before taking the next step.

Don't get me wrong, I know exactly where I'm going, and things are lining up, making it very obvious what's next. At the same time, there have been challenges that have been so potent and profound, I've decided to sit back and ponder for a moment.

I believe we are challenged the most when we are ready for exponential growth. I believe we are triggered when we have some healing to do. And I believe that *everything*, and I mean everything, is a reflection of who we are.

The healing that has taken place over the last three weeks has me feeling so new and... exposed. My senses are heightened and my psychic abilities are emerging into a new but very familiar level of attunement. It's like I can see what's next, and now it's time to just jump in and do it with a level of consciousness that is, well, up-leveled.

I have been toying with this idea of girl empowerment and the elevation of the Divine Feminine for quite some time—years actually. But you cannot fully move forward until you recognize why these "callings to do something" are so potent to your own existence. And here's why:

Your calling is always, and I mean always, a deep healing opportunity for yourself, which in turn heals the collective, which is really why you are here.

And we needn't wait to be "perfect" in order to "do our work" or help others. Quite the contrary. We put ourselves out there as we are and lovingly use our tools to heal ourselves while helping others find their way.

I've taken thousands of yoga classes, been a part of hundreds of teleseminars, sat in circle with many people, held space for individuals, and cried many tears of release, regret, and joy.

But it has been over fifteen years since I sat, on a beach, by myself, and asked myself and the Higher Powers that Be... what is my highest calling? It's been that long since I sat in silence for more than an hour of meditation. That long since I booked a flight anywhere, by myself with no idea what was next.

It's been that long since I said, "I'm outta here and I'm tuning out for a bit. Forgive me, but my soul needs this." I've been in a survival mode for over six years and before that, I was asleep at the helm of my own life. This yoga thing woke me up over thirteen years ago, and it continues to peel away the layers of my own being so I can continue to be more, rest more, see more, and witness truth and love in action. For real.

I have been called to live my life in a very different way than I was raised. Asked to be a little different or unique, as my daughters say. I've always lived my life like this. And the Caribbean Sea holds my heart and soul. I'm not sure why, or if I will ever know why, but I just know it is truth.

After all the turmoil in the planets and astrological mayhem, which is really mystical cohesiveness disguised, I feel like this trip to Tulum has been divinely dropped into my lap. I told myself I wouldn't take any more trips unless they were to a high-energy vortex spot, and I'm thinking I may be dropping into one, just in time for the new moon in Gemini.

Everything I'm reading and studying is talking about new paradigms, uplifting consciousness, and big changes. And this New Moon on June 16 is about delivering just that. All the subsequent eclipses and potent full moons have been orchestrating our own personal illuminations while awakening those who are open to it. Mostly everyone I know is experiencing this on some level... there are just some who are conscious to it and some who are not.

I'm off the grid for a few days, ya'll. You may see a few Instagram posts from the beach but just know... it's time. It's time to up-level and I'm doing just that. I'm just going to recharge in Tulum first so I can be of complete service to the Divine when I return.

See you on the other side!

New Moon—Winter Solstice

You know, I will never pretend to know everything, not ever. Because I know better!

However, I will say this: I do know and am very familiar with my intuitive intelligence. And lately, it's been speaking so damn loud! I mean, I've heard so much lately that sometimes, I try to distract or dramatize. You know what I mean? It's much easier, sometimes, to be busy than it is to fess up, clear out, get real and get moving!

Right?

Well, guess what? The gig is up. There's no more playing around. It's time to come out of hiding; well, at least you should start thinking about it anyway. Personally, I feel like I'm now down to my final layers and, let me say, they are ready to be pulled off! Although... technically I have until the Spring equinox to fully "come out."

I don't know what you're doing, but I'm going to make sure I'm sitting, breathing, being and surrounding myself with those souls I find most resonance with. Why? Because it's dark and I feel safe when I sit, hear my breath, and am surrounded by energy that pulses with mine and creates a balance of support and love.

This is the darkest night of the year. Some are even calling it the collective "dark night of the soul"—when all is revealed and all is illuminated beyond the darkness. And it has been dark, hasn't it? Not just on an individual level but on a global one. Just sit for a moment with everything that has happened.

It's been dark.

But this season is such a beautiful time of incubation, recreation and recalibration. It's time to go inward and if you're not doing that, I promise you, soon enough the Universe will see to it that you will. Why?

Because it's important, it's important to know where you're going in this fast-paced world. It's important to know what you value. What you love. What you live for and what you would die for. I believe this is a collective thing that each one of us is feeling on some level, whether we choose to be awake to it or not. The Universe has come a knocking and it's time to wake up.

It's important to realign so you can hear this calling, but in order to do that, sometimes you just have to sit. Sit and allow, sit and pray, sit and observe, sit and breathe. Sit and see what happens when you do nothing. See what happens when you rest. Whenever I sit and rest, life shows up. When I get off the treadmill and spin my internal dhristi back behind my eyes, my vision is clear and life really shows up. And, most often, in ways I know I have been intending but maybe not exactly as I had thought. Either way, the path is illuminated and I can choose to follow it or not.

You see, the darkness is necessary for growth, for clarity, for illumination. And when you sit in it long enough you just know which way to go.

This is the time, ya'll. Time to sit in empty presence and just be with what is happening. Pull it in and then let what is unnecessary drop away... make space for breath, for clarity, for connection and for a sure-foot forward.

Soon enough the light of day will be streaming into your sleepy eyes. But for now, sit in the darkness and listen. Listen to the beat of your heart, the whisper of your soul, the calling of your intuitive intelligence. Get ready to act confidently... it's time.

New Reality

The 11/11 New Moon in Scorpio opened up a portal that we all had (and still have) an opportunity to walk through—a portal that would support us in thinking differently, dissolving our burdens, and observing ourselves as we are, in the Now.

The present astrological events of this full moon in Gemini and Saturn-Neptune square bring it all home. When we entered this New Moon energy, we came in as one thing and are now BEing released as quite another.

This release may happen for us consciously or unconsciously; we may surrender willingly or we may put up a fight. Either way, the cosmos have a way of aligning things for us whether we like it or not. Over the years, I have learned to pay just enough attention and, given the opportunity, comply.

Everything is lined up for a huge shift in consciousness individually and, if enough of us are open to this shift, globally. Big changes CAN happen if enough of us drop in and listen, and then open to expand into a new reality.

Just this week I was driving from the East Bay in the early morning hours and I looked at the Western sky and saw La Luna. The Eastern sky was still dark, so She was like a beacon, big and bright as ever. I felt like I was driving into a mural, a mirage, with the Bay Bridge lights, city skyline and mountains as a backdrop.

And then I remembered—oh yeah, this is my life.

The beauty, the magic, the connections, the love, the grief, the not knowing, the loneliness, the yearning for partnership, the gratitude, the freedom, the hard work, the surrender, the infinite truth. It's a reality I created for the evolution of my soul—which, I am constantly reminded, is a lifelong job.

Guru Brahma, Guru Vishnu, Guru devo Maheshwara,
Guru Sakshat, Param Brahma, Tasmai shri Guravay namah

It wasn't too long ago that I was in fear, trying to stand on my own two feet and create the life I had longed for; not long at all. And here I stand in it completely.

I stepped into my a reality once in 1992 when I drove my car across the country and moved away from my family of origin and set up shop in San Diego. Then again when I moved with my then husband, from San Diego to Portland where I thought the "householder" had to live. Both times, I gave birth to my lovely angels. Again, when I signed divorce papers on 11/11/11. And again on 11/13/12, when I moved from Portland to San Francisco to start a new life.

My realities used to consist of living in an old paradigm of lack and limit. Guilt, shame and grief ruled my actions. An illusion that I had to do it all or it wouldn't get done. A misconception that if I let my heart out to be held, it would be trampled.

Along this journey, these patterns and delusions served and protected me, somehow. But over time, and with evolution and expansion, one by one, they dropped from my way of being. Without them, though, I never would have gotten here—which is open, vulnerable, raw and in love with this life.

Every step of the way was a current state of "reality" that was challenging and full of karmic lessons and observation. Now, I am on the brink of a new reality. I always get excited when this happens.

The truth is, you are living new realities all the time—you are evolving all the time. You can shift and create new realities multiple times in one lifetime.

I was once told, "*The stability that you desire cannot become frozen or static. The more you create, the quicker things move through your life. This is creating; not manipulating, but creating.*"

So I ask you, in this full moon energy, what new reality would you like to create? What needs to shift so you can step into that magic you once believed in as a kid? What needs to be released during this full moon and bonus, Saturn-Neptune square?

The cosmos want to know and so do I, honestly. I ask you to observe your patterns with the deepest self-love and compassion and explore those questions. Ask yourself what served you in your last reality and what can you let go of in order to leap into your new one. I know you know what it is; now just do it.

October Moons

I have to be honest and tell you that I am bit excited about the planetary shifts happening right now. I was feeling a little overwhelmed and then I remembered that my feet were firmly planted in the ground and I really had nothing to worry about. I might beam away, but I won't blow away.

From what I gather, here's the deal:

We've got intensely moving planets up there, milling around to create a re-alignment of sorts for us all.

Mercury is now in retrograde, which means going inward, even backward if you will, for a review of your past. It's in the water sign of Scorpio, which is about your feelings and intimate relationships. Hmmmmm...

Whenever Mercury goes into retrograde, its focus is on communication. So this particular retrograde is about your feelings about a past relationship and how to heal what is still wounded so you can move forward into the light of this full moon.

But hang on...

When Mercury moves back into the sign of Libra on 10/10 (interesting) you will have a greater understanding of your relationships and how to heal imbalances in your life... this in relation to your feelings about love.

This is only two days after the blood moon, lunar eclipse in Aries... the first fire sign of the zodiac.

But hang on...

When Mercury went into hiding, it was energized by the Fire Trine of Mars, Jupiter and Uranus... which is like taking all this information and putting into a magnifying glass of your future... resulting in miracles.

You actually SEE your Big Picture with clarity and depth... and you recognize what needs to be burned or let go of in order to move toward that.

Now, on to the full moon lunar eclipse in Aries... Hang on to your hats!

Aries is the first sign of the Zodiac, which is pretty bold, leading the way with courage and zing—all formidable and fiery and stuff. Makes me think of Durga, to be honest.

So, when this moon is full and then is eclipsed, just after the Uranus trine and during Mercury retrograde, what I'm gathering is this:

Whatever you have been holding onto... let go now, or you could run the risk of being dragged. A story, a relationship that isn't working, whatever is draining you, you must let go now. And courageously... knowing that you will be carried into the miracle you are dreaming into your reality.

That means no more story telling, no more waiting until later, no more putting it off. That means... now.

Eclipses want you to break free from old stuff, and Uranus expects out-of-the-blue haphazardness; however, Mercury in retrograde is giving you the space to reflect, renew, realign, redesign, recalibrate, all those re-words, before moving forward.

I think of it as walking into the magic mirror—the mirror that I have been watching with my heart forever; the mirror that turns to liquid when you step one foot into it; the mirror that has been summoning me for years to trust, to open, to love, to dream it into reality.

You know the one, right?

As you walk through that space, as you step boldly forward, watch where you are going, maybe take one glance back, bow in gratitude for it all and then jump on in, leaving it all behind.

Purification

When I heard, at the beginning of April, that the New Moon was in Aries, pushing us to move into our extreme, most empowered self, I got so excited! Then when I heard that just fifteen days later, we were going to experience a Full Moon ON a Lunar Eclipse, I got a little nervous. When I read that following that Full Moon, there was going to be a New Moon that coincided with a Solar Eclipse, I started looking for shelter. Then, when I read that the Cardinal Grand Cross was sitting in the middle of these two Eclipses, honestly, I wanted to grab a drink. Crazy chaos out in those planets. And nothing we can control.

I haven't studied astrology... I haven't had to. I have the best friends who inform me when things are about to go way wacky. This one was big, though. I could feel this one. I felt it coming on before it happened. And to be honest, I did want to grab a drink. I wanted to hunker down, have lots of sex, sleep, eat and just hope we would all survive afterward.

But I didn't. I mean, that's what most of the world does in times of chaos. We drink, we smoke, we have sex, we distract. We busy ourselves so we don't have to feel into the pain of our lives. Or live with the decision we made that isn't working for us. We get all up in everyone else's business as well, because it's a hell of a lot easier to tell them what to do than it is to look at or clean up our own mess.

Nope, not this time. This time I said... "let's purify more and FEEL into the pain, the heartache, the longing, the loneliness, the hurt. Let's get in there... clean and clear, and face it." I mean why not, you're here. Can't we just wake up to our lives, already? It's not an easy job but we are truly the only ones who can do it. We keep looking outside ourselves for help... for guidance... but the only place to look is in that pile of shit you keep ignoring because it smells so bad.

Here's what worries me... there are so many distractions out there that, if we're not careful, we will become so numb to pain that we'll morph into robots. Little robots who can't formulate a sentence, who can't look at someone in the eyes and can't sit up straight because they are too used to looking down into an electronic device. We'll have our phones tethered to our waist, a bluetooth in our ear and eventually glasses on that hook us up to the Internet in a blink of an eye... literally.

I'm sorry, but I think—and I could be mistaken—that we were born to feel. And to feel deeply. So, then why do we humans keep creating things that keep us from doing that? We have to stop.

So... we purify.

And since the body we walk around with all day, every day is so dense, we may as well start there. Purifying the body. How do we do it?

Move your body.

Well, we start with moving it. I mean, we are a society that sits so damn much it's almost ridiculous. I read an article about ten years ago that said that most people of Sicily actually live to be 100 years old because they spend their lives outside, tending to their land. Moving their bodies.

Watch what you eat.

Because anyone can run, bike, sweat in yoga, and do a 1,000 sit-ups but it doesn't mean anything if you're putting crap into your body. You'll just have a food hangover and feel worse about yourself. I have come to subscribe to this. If you cleanse once... I mean one really big, huge cleanse, and then eat food that will nourish your body and not contaminate it, you should be just fine. What does that look like?

Well, the list could go on and on... no sugar, no dairy, no white stuff, no caffeine, no alcohol and no processed food. For the love of God, no fast food and no GMOS. What the hell does that leave us, people? Really? When you're only feeding yourself, it's pretty easy but what about when you have two kids who go to school with kids who still bring half-eaten McDonald's to school and have a pack of Hostess doughnuts for dessert. That's where it gets tricky, to be sure. Not to mention if your spouse, partner or ex-husband doesn't exactly see eye-to-eye with your food choices. So I say, do a massive cleanse and then be good! Trust me, after you cleanse really well, you won't want to eat any of that stuff.

Green juice... every single day. And I don't mean the store-bought ones. I mean, you make it yourself or have it made at a juice bar or bought from a reputable, local company where you can pick it up just after it's made and it only lasts two days in the refrigerator. Sure, it's expensive but it will cost you less in medical bills.

Turmeric kills everything. So does apple cider vinegar. Put those on lots of food. Buy local, organic food when you can. And when you can't, read the labels and do your best. Drink water. Educate your kids about why you are so intense about this process—and why you give in sometimes, too.

Purify the mind.

Did you know that we have about seventy thousand thoughts a day? And, of those seventy thousand thoughts, about 1 percent of them are new thoughts. That means that we are running on a program based on old thoughts... almost all day long. Not only that, but we only take about fifty thousand breaths in one day. So that means we have more thoughts in a day than we do breaths. That sucks.

So how do we slow those thoughts down? We breathe slower without doing anything else while we are breathing. We watch the thoughts and we begin the self-inquiry process of discernment. *Is this thought helpful? Is it kind and loving? Is it mine? Is this a pattern? Is the pattern working for me?*

We run at warp speed, to be sure, and, honestly, I think we are all working on these patterns that, if we really stopped to look at them, we would realize are taking us away from what we want instead of moving us forward.

Look at what you are watching on TV.

Violent, dramatic programs... not so good. The news... for the love of God, NO! We are drawn to drama and fear-based programs to... distract. What are you watching? Is it filling you up? How is it making you feel? What are you dreaming about afterward? If you must watch TV, pick only those programs that offer you solid information or make you feel good inside and fill you up.

Computer time.

Oh, that lovely, shiny box that promised us our life would become more efficient. Just like the microwave did. A devil in disguise. This thing is an evil necessity, so treat it as such. Do what you need to do and then be done. Create transition time in between this "work" and bedtime. Look at how much time you are spending on it and only do what is necessary. Set boundaries. This is about your energy and how you are using it. You're not moving your body if you are on your computer or hunched over your phone.

Quick death.

Get up every forty-five minutes and move! Then at the end of the day, shut it down and read, practice yoga, write, make love. Anything that rewires the energy input into your eyeballs and through your fingers.

Your phone.

Ok... super-fun ring tones, tweet sounds and vibrational noises are unique to each individual. Whatever works, so you know whether the call coming in is important or not. However, it's not important for you to answer your phone right away. It's really not. Let the thing sit for a minute after the bell and then go for it. We are programmed to jump when that bell goes off. Stop it. I remember reading something about how fireman get all messed up in the head being woken up by those alarms and having to be prepared and ready to go in the blink of an eye. This is no different. Except... newsflash... there's no fire you have to put out right this second.

Your friends.

Who are you hanging out with? What are their beliefs? What do they like to do? How positive are they about the world around them? How do you feel around them? And this may shift over time because you are changing. Let's be honest, sometimes it's just time to switch up your circle of friends. And everyone will be better for it. Look at how much energy you are inputting into the relationship and ask yourself if it is imbalanced. If it is, you have the responsibility to make it right.

Then, of course, there is purification of the heart. Now I had no idea that this was a book but, apparently, it is. I have never picked it up, on purpose. I wanted to formulate my own thing here. This is what I came up with.

The breath.

We were given this breath the second we were born and it's the last thing we do before we pass on to the next life. The breath is the element of the heart. So then how do we go through so many of our days not taking gratitude for the breath? Not taking long, deep breaths. It's a necessity for clarity, for health and for life. It creates space between thought and reaction. And you want that so you react from a place that is laced in truth and love... not patterns.

Love.

Who are you loving? How are you loving? Are you showing them gratitude and appreciation? Are you loving them as they are and not trying to change them? Are you telling them that you love them without expecting anything in return. Random acts of kindness... unnecessary love notes. That's what I say!

Forgive.

What's in there darkening your light? What is it? Someone hurt you, yes. We all get hurt. It's part of life. It is life. Now what? Do you want to hold onto it and talk about it some more? How does it make you feel? There are many quotes on forgiveness, and here's the deal: The only person you are hurting when you don't forgive is yourself. That's it. I don't care what it is... forgive it. You needn't forget it... just forgive. Without understanding, without attachment to an outcome, without even needing to tell that person you are forgiving them. Just be right with it in your own heart.

In times of chaos it's so easy to get caught up in the patterns, the energy and the feeling that is swirling around you. Don't do it. Stop, drop and breathe. Sit. Be still. Observe what you are doing and how you are showing up. That is the only job you have. From there you can function from a place that is real and true. Everything else is someone else's path and you want to be on your own... pure and simple.

Shedding

The Year of the Snake: shedding the old and moving into the new with faith and trust. The New Moon, new beginnings, releasing of old patterns. Seems easy enough, right?

But how tightly do you hold onto old patterns, ideas and even people just because it is easy and comfortable? This may show up as a repeated circumstance, a familiar argument or even chronic pain or anxiety. However it shows up, it's stagnating energy and it needs to flow... now.

What does it feel like when you are getting ready to shed an old dimension of yourself? It is consistent tremors through the body. It's loss of sleep and loss of breath. It's that feeling you may feel just before you jump off a cliff or out of an airplane. Scary as hell!

You're scared because most often you don't know what's on the other side. Most often you don't know if you will be alone, judged, broke, hurt or exposed. You just don't know. So to jump from complacency to the unknown is quite a courageous leap.

You may even sabotage your jump. You are in that stage of "in-between," experiencing the old and the new all at once. That is oh so confusing! In the physical reality you are saying, "YES, I'm ready for this up-level in my career, relationship, environment, spiritual connection." But on a deeper level you are so afraid to let go of what you know, so you sabotage.

Your old patterns of blame, isolation, and frustration rear their head and keep you rooted in the old. I mean, what would happen if you actually made millions on your idea or your artistry? What would happen if you actually moved to a new town and knew no one? And you had to find a new coffee shop and new way to work? What would happen then?

And what would happen if you actually experienced a love greater than you could even imagine for yourself? I mean, really? You would have to be totally exposed and open to someone else's judgments; it is easier to isolate, right?

Wrong.

Most importantly, what would it feel like to be guided by the hand of God in every moment? Could you trust that? Could you feel it and become it in every moment? How often would you turn your back and say, "No thanks, I know better."

How do you move into a place of trusting completely?

You embody compassion... grace... gratitude... breath... vulnerability... letting go of the need to know it all or be right. Because as you move into the new you, what you knew, what you know now is misaligned with whom you are becoming. In fact, what you know now may have been the very thing that has kept you from true momentum forward.

So, what do you do? You breathe. You examine with love what is in front of you. You see things as an infant sees things, with innocence and curiosity. However, the truth is that you are NOT an infant and you have walls, patterns and old hurts, so curiosity can be challenging.

Because why? Because you will be triggered big time! Several times a day perhaps. And most likely, by the people who are showing up to show you the way.

So what do you do? You give in and you listen with a heart that might be beating and blood that might be boiling, and you cool it all down with the love in your heart. So, if your heart has been hurt, this may be painful. But the fire in your belly is what purifies the heart. The breath you take in stokes the fire to purify the hurt in the heart. It allows you to truly see what is real with love.

You watch your actions closely. Are they moving you forward or back? You witness your thoughts. It's like you're watching a movie and you get to change the outcome of each frame or chapter based on your willingness to be open to the unknown outcome of your choice.

Will you perhaps trip and fall? Sure, and perhaps quite often. Now, it's like you are a child learning to walk. A new walk, a new path. The old path wasn't working... it WORKED for where you were at the time but you are on a new path now.

Scary... yes. But I can tell you that complacency has no place in the healing of our planet. It's okay to retreat, recoil and fall back into old ways every now and again. You're human... it's part of the experience. Take a rest in complacency, it is comfortable. A snake doesn't rip its skin off and say, "I'm ready!" A snake sheds it in just the right time.

Be confident that when you're ready to come out again, you will be supported by individuals, circumstance, and of course, by God, as you move into this new version of yourself. Be a child again and trust the world. It is here for your benefit and your exploration of your soul.

Shine

With all this planetary shifting happening, it's been hard, honestly, to focus. Have you felt it? It's as though the ground has been unsettled underneath my feet. You might expect forward motion but, instead, all I want to do is hunker down and take a nap. And for those of you who know me... you know that I am not a napper.

My body has been tired and my mind has been... alive. Even my dreams have been so vivid it's as though I'm living in another dimension while I'm sleeping. So, yes, I've been super sleepy.

But life keeps marching forward... and all this letting go, affirming, praying, purifying and moving my body didn't produce the results I thought it would. I thought I would feel light, airy, free and weightless. I was waiting for a choir of angels to sing, "Alleluia... here it is... go this way!" But that hasn't happened yet.

Well, that is, until today.

Today, Easter Sunday, I was blessed to spend a few hours with the remarkable Tina Malia, right here in Fairfax at Sol Studios. She is a connected, powerful being who has the voice of an angel. I play her music in my class, sing to her music in the morning, and "My Practice Playlist" has her voice all over it.

Today, during her Artist's Salon, inspiration was born. Thank God, because I was really scared for a moment. It really came down to one simple statement, one divine moment, one little chat I had after the session with a random man by the name of Wolf and his artist friend Ian... but here's the process...

Tina made many statements that really resonated with me. So much so, that I could have been up there saying the same exact things. (I do on many occasions, actually.)

She related her song writing and performing to a balance of art and science. She said that it's hard for her to be completely vulnerable, but she pushes herself to do it because she knows on some level, somewhere, someone is healing because of her words and songs. She said she likes to tell stupid jokes because it's more important that everyone feel welcome and like a family rather than her preaching about spirituality and music. She made a point to mention that she is no better than anyone else in the room and that we are all just reflections of each other. She said that every song she writes tells a story and ends with a resolution.

She said that she cannot possibly give her manager a set list two weeks prior to her concert. She has to wake up that morning, feel the venue, feel the crowd and then she can come up with her set list. And she said that, in times of despair, Jai Uttal told her to chant Ram until she felt better. She did it for three years before she saw the light within herself.

I was crying, listening to her. What a beautiful reflection for me, sitting there with my two daughters who are enthralled by her beauty, authenticity and artistry.

I, too, chanted Ram, 108 times for days, weeks and months, through tears until I found the light. I tell stupid jokes in my class just for fun. I, too, never plan a class; it just comes. I relate all of my yoga sessions as a storytelling, because every movement opens up a part of the body to healing—to ending—to an opening. I too make sure people see my imperfections because, guess what? I'm not perfect; no one is. And far be it from me to preach as if I am.

I am an extraordinary light, to be sure, but I, too, feel uncomfortable sitting in that amazing light sometimes.

The thing that inspired me the most and brought me to tears in Good Earth today was a look into my life and how beautiful it is. And how I created it all based on my belief in myself and in God. I felt so full and complete because, through her, I saw myself.

I bow with deep gratitude as I let go of so much pain from my past and finally see myself in my highest light. Sometimes our words have to come before we believe it ourselves. We have to say things first, to trick the brain into believing what the heart knows to be true.

This is the simple message. Are you ready? It's time to step into your light. It's time to see your most amazing self on this planet. I have been saying it for years and have been, yes, living it. But the funny thing is... the more you live it the more you become it. And then the light isn't this flickering little light that lives in your heart; it is something that precedes you for miles. It's something that people feel before you walk into the room. It's something that is infinite and has to be shared because you can't possibly hold it in.

Yeah... that's where I'm going with all this. I'm "doing the thing." It's time to get some new sunglasses. You in?

Solar Eclipse Magic

Oh, my Goddess... anyone else out there feeling the planets shifting as if they were shifting inside your own body? If you don't, just sit still for a minute, you will. I mean... we begin to recover from the aftermath of a FULL MOON LUNAR ECLIPSE and are just about to enter into a NEW MOON SOLAR ECLIPSE while MERCURY IS IN RETROGRADE!

To add to all the fun, the Solar Eclipse is in Scorpio, which means a magnifying glass on sensuality, sexuality, and primal instincts. This is big and literally could be quite orgasmic. But hang on, Mercury is still in retrograde so just chill for a second.

There are six planets creating a T-square (it looks like a perfect triangle really) in the midst of this New Moon Eclipse. What does this mean?

Breakthroughs. Astounding, supernatural breakthroughs. Yes, that is correct. This word came to me in a reading AFTER I called it out as the theme for the week. But I am not surprised; no, I actually believe it all. I have always known that the Universe supports me; it's just that sometimes I want things to roll a little smoother than they do.

I liken this sort of energy to the anticipation of being shot out of a cannon. In some circles, it has been described as an "uber" rebirth: one that is intense and empowering, one that will change the course of your life as much as you will allow.

My suggestion? Allow the energy to have its way. There's no use in kicking and screaming. It won't do you any good; you may get dragged if you resist.

I don't know about you but I have felt every bit of this one. And here's what I have to say:

Thank you Universe for breaking my computer for just a hot minute so I could be responsible and back it up before it was too late.

Thank you Universe for backing me into a corner so I had no other recourse but to ask for support and guidance.

Thank you Universe for illuminating the areas of my life that no longer serve me without strangling me or rendering me injured.

Thank you Universe for the reminder of how potent and beneficial breath, stillness, and transparency can be in a moment.

Thank you Universe for dropping every unresolved issue into my lap in the last two weeks so I can finally let them go with fierce compassion.

Thank you Universe for slamming on the brakes of my own plans so I could dive more deeply into the relationship I have with my daughters.

Thank you Universe for ripping open every scab that I thought was healed. Apparently, they needed more medicine.

Thank you mostly for the reminder that I am an embodiment of light and love and that everything I ask for I am deserved to receive.

Thank you for reminding me that in one breath I can receive all the space I need to change courses and to see what is real while loving it all.

I really, really appreciate every bit of magic you have offered up in this magnificent display of mystical orchestration. You do your work so simply, so effortlessly, so eloquently... I wonder sometimes why I doubt you. Why I look to anything but you and inside my own transcendent body for guidance.

Buckle up... set your intentions... be ready for a magical, mystical show. It's called your life.

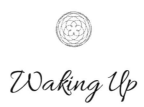

Waking Up

I was watching the full moon the other night with a friend and felt very small. We were sitting on a hilltop, looking over the cities of Tiburon, Sausalito, San Francisco, and Oakland. The bay was shrouded in clouds and fog but still shone so brightly. The cloud cover added such a sense of majestic mystery to this eclipse that I felt like I should have been paying an admission fee to someone for the show. This show, which I call my life. This movie that is full of infinite lessons, challenges, initiations, triumphs and epic transitions. This box office blockbuster.

I was looking up at the stars, and all the planes flying around in the air, going somewhere. And all the cars driving up and down Highway 101, headed somewhere.

Did they know there was an eclipse? Did they know the moon was rising in all her glory? Did they know that there was a really cool event about to happen in the sky that wouldn't happen for another eighteen years? Did they understand just how small their issues were? Did they get it? You know, that we are all one, watching the same moon and the same sky?

Or where they overwhelmed in their own drama? In their own story? In their own capsule of reality going... somewhere? I sat there staring at the moon and I asked my friend, "If you could wish one thing on this eclipse night, what would it be? What would you like to see on the other side of this moon?" He said simply, "I want more people to wake up. I just want more people to wake up."

My heart stopped, literally. Yes... that is what the world needs—more people to wake up; to remember that this is but a dream that we are creating; to know that we GET to live this life any way we want; to know that every person on this planet is a soul living their karmic destiny; that everyone is someone to somebody.

The reality is that most people on this planet are sleeping. They are sleeping through their lives, through intimate connections, and through their lessons. Sometimes I look around and get so dismayed and sad, I cry. I witness so much unconsciousness and such an obvious loss of connection. I witness entitlement, separation, greed, and an overall sense of lack.

I have to be honest here and say, every single day, I thank God I do what I do. I thank God that I chose to share this love of yoga because in my field, at least people are trying to wake up. I pray, along with my sweet friend, that more people just wake the hell up. Because it's exhausting to hit the snooze button over and over again. It actually messes up your REM, you know.

I know it can be equally exhausting being awake through your life, too. I know; I get it. Seemingly it is easier to sleep it off, medicate (rather than meditate), distract and blame outside influence, claiming that there's "nothing we can do." It is so much easier to stay asleep. Yeah, I get it.

But the truth is that once you wake up, yeah, you're in. And the reality is that if you even try and go back to sleep, you're in for a lot of suffering, confusion and unnecessary back pedaling. So why don't you just succumb and wake the hell up?

Get off your high horse and get in the game of life where it's messy, and chaotic, and not so timely and epic and magic and completely unpredictable. That's where we wake up. When things get a little hairy. And for once, just once, can you sit in it and be in it? Can you not avoid it, avert from it, distract yourself with some pathetic story of times gone by or fantasy of the future, and just be in it?

Be in the awakeness... in the reality of awakening. Because, truth be told, being awake is amazing. And lovely, and the best amusement park ride ever. It's twisting and turning and dropping you down to take you right back up.

Even when I close my eyes, I still feel every single bit of this ride. And I love it, every single bit.

I might cry at disappointment, get angry at injustice, and become frustrated and impatient when I think I know better. But I can honestly say I am awake. I might not "get it right" in every moment. I might not speak with my yogi-tongue in every exchange.

But I can honestly say I am awake.

I see.

I feel.

I try.

I practice.

I fall.

I get messy.

I say, wake up people. Wake up to this epic journey. Step out of your phones, your distractions and other peoples' stories and look up. Look at the stars, at the moon and at the sky. Get up high on a mountaintop and see how small you really are. Look in the mirror and recognize your beauty, your grace, your gifts—this miracle you call you.

Stop wasting your time on sleeping, on blaming, on separating. Wake up to the reality of Oneness. Wake up to the reality of Now. Wake up to the reality of Love.

Period.

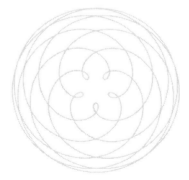

About The Author

Dana Damara has embraced yoga as a lifestyle both on and off the mat. Through her children, writing, and creation of meaningful relationships with the community around her, Dana has facilitated that power of soulfulness and spiritual awakening through yoga, both for others and herself.

Damara moves and breathes with the breath of the Universe. She thrives in the face of adversity, understanding that everything that happens to us actually happens *for* us. She dances with meditation and yoga, knowing that this practice alone helps to protect the mind from distractions that keep us from our most vibrant path.

She is guardian of the soul... bringing you to new heights of awareness with her craft and passionate flair. She is a rock, with soft edges and authentic vulnerabilities. Do not mistake her kindness for ignorance; she is SPIRIT and can see truth. She has shed her many veils. She was born with the power to see through your exterior to your soul.

She exudes a balance of strength, vulnerability, openness and drive. She is a mover and a shaker and she will shake your ego until you let your soul out to be heard. Her courage isn't to be feared, though, as her heart holds the world in its own hands. Her heart is a magnet, drawing those to her who seek more in life than the mundane.

Dana comes alive when you bear witness to your own power and strength– as she is nothing more than a guide and a life long change queen. She will take you on a journey to your Self many times over and you will never look back as you shed your own ego.

Her secrets? EQUANIMITY, TRUST, INTUITION and UNCONDI-TIONAL LOVE. She offers these gifts to you through this book, as well as YOGISYNERGY, YOGIS4YOGA, her classes, workshops and her accredited yoga teacher training/spiritual development program. Come and play with this spiritual warrior...your life will shift immediately.

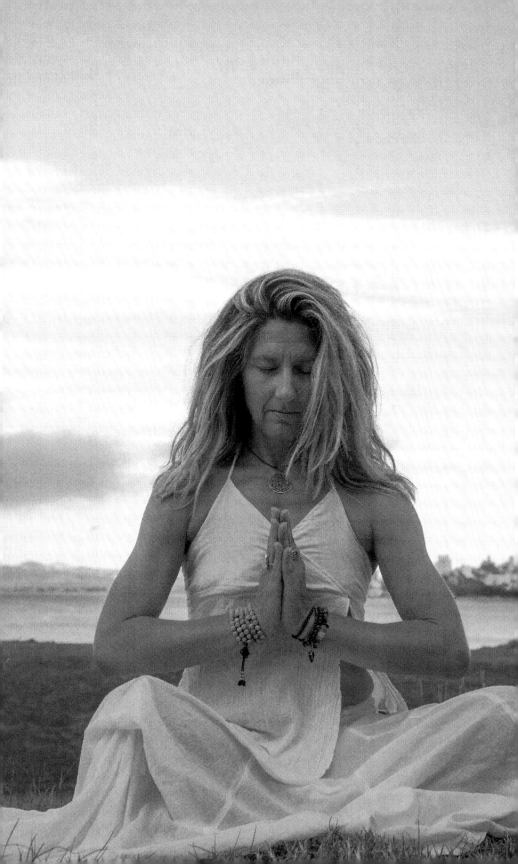

Made in the USA
Middletown, DE
06 March 2020